8th Edition

Treat Your Own
Back

Robin McKenzie CNZM, OBE, FCSP (Hon.) FNZSP (Hon.), Dip MDT, Dip MT

Spinal Publications New Zealand Ltd
1 Alexander Road, PO Box 2026
Raumati Beach, New Zealand
Email: enquiries@spinalpublications.co.nz
Telephone: ++ 64 4 299-7020

ISBN-10: 0-9582692-3-8

ISBN-13: 978-0-9582692-3-0

Edited by Autumnwood Editing, www.autumnwood.biz

Designed by Next Communications, Inc.

Photography by Tony Kellaway and TKA Photography

First Edition first published in 1980 by New Zealand University Press/Price Milburn

Second Edition January 1981 Spinal Publications New Zealand Ltd

Third Edition	September, 1985
Fourth Edition	March, 1988
Fifth Edition	May, 1992
Sixth Edition	April, 1993
Seventh Edition	January, 1997
Eight Edition	July, 2006

Acknowledgements

Hugh Price, an old schoolmate of mine, suffered from acute and severe recurrent back pain for many years. In 1978, after one particularly agonizing bout, he came to see me and I showed him how to straighten out his bent back and stop his pain in only twenty-four hours. He recovered so quickly and was so impressed that he said I should write a book telling people how this could be done. I replied that I was too busy in my practice and could never take that sort of time; besides, I had no literary skills. He said to me that if I gave him my detailed patient instruction sheets he would turn them into a book for me.

Hugh was a principal in the publishing company of Price Milburn, so he had the skills and expertise. The result was the first edition of this book printed in 1979. It has since been rewritten and updated over several revised editions, and has been translated into seventeen languages.

I have received many valuable suggestions for inclusion in this edition from senior faculty of the McKenzie Institute International. In particular I must thank Colin Davies, Robert Medcalf, Stephen May and Hugh Murray. Treat Your Own Back has become the world's biggest-selling back book of all time and both you and I have to thank Hugh Price and the others for this, the eighth edition.

About the Author

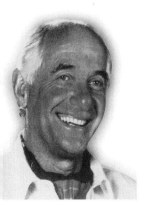

Robin McKenzie was born in Auckland, New Zealand, in 1931. After attending Wairarapa College, he enrolled in the New Zealand School of Physiotherapy, from which he graduated in 1952. Since 1953, when he commenced private practice in Wellington, New Zealand, he has specialized in the treatment of spinal disorders.

During the 1960s Robin McKenzie developed his own examination and treatment methods and is now recognized internationally as an authority on the diagnosis and treatment of low back pain. He has lectured internationally and, to give some indication of the success of the system of treatment he has developed, the McKenzie Method of mechanical diagnosis and therapy is now taught and practiced worldwide. In the United States, the United Kingdom, Ireland and in New Zealand, the McKenzie Method is the preferred treatment of choice among physiotherapists for back problems.

In June 2004 the *ADVANCE* for physical therapists and physical therapy assistants in the United States, published the results of a survey sent to a random sampling of 320 physical therapists from the orthopaedic section of the American Physical Therapy Association. The therapists were asked which physical therapists or physicians of all time had had the biggest influence in their thinking or performance in orthopaedic physical therapy. The clinician voted the number one most influential was Robin McKenzie.

The success of the McKenzie Method has attracted intense interest from researchers in various parts of the world, and it is one of the most studied diagnostic and treatment systems for back pain at the present time. An extensive list of scientific studies carried out worldwide demonstrates the efficacy and importance of the diagnostic process and the treatment system. If you are interested in reading more about this, go to www.mckenziemdt.org.

To ensure the orderly development of education and research into the methods devised by Robin McKenzie, doctors and physiotherapists involved in the teaching process formed the McKenzie Institute International in 1982. The Institute is a not-for-profit organization with headquarters in New Zealand. Robin McKenzie was elected the first president of the Institute.

Robin McKenzie has published in the *New Zealand Medical Journal* and contributed to many authoritative texts on back problems. He is the author of six books: *Treat Your Own Back, Treat Your Own Neck, Seven Steps to a Pain Free Life,* (2000), *The Lumbar Spine: Mechanical Diagnosis & Therapy* (1981 and 2003), *The Cervical and Thoracic Spine: Mechanical Diagnosis & Therapy* (1990 and 2006), and *The Human Extremities: Mechanical Diagnosis & Therapy* (2000).

The contributions Robin McKenzie has made to the understanding and treatment of musculoskeletal problems have been internationally recognized. In 1982 he was made an Honorary Life Member of the American Physical Therapy Association "in recognition of distinguished and meritorious service to the art and science of physical therapy and to the welfare of mankind."

In 1983 he was elected to membership of the International Society for the Study of the Lumbar Spine. In 1984 he was made a Fellow of the American Back Society and in 1985 he was awarded an Honorary Fellowship of the New Zealand Society of Physiotherapists. In 1987 he was made an Honorary Life Member of the New Zealand Manipulative Therapists Association and in 1990 an Honorary Fellow of the Chartered Society of Physiotherapists in the United Kingdom.

In the 1990 Queen's Birthday Honours, he was made an Officer of the Most Excellent Order of the British Empire (OBE). In the New Year Honours 2000, Her Majesty Queen Elizabeth II appointed Robin McKenzie to be a Companion of the New Zealand Order of Merit (CNZM).

Chapter 4: *Understanding the McKenzie Method* 30
    Aim of the Exercises 30
    Effect on Pain Intensity and Location 31
        Centralization 33
    How to Know if You Are Exercizing Correctly 35

Chapter 5: *The Exercise Program* 36
    Exercise 1: Lying Face Down 36
    Exercise 2: Lying Face Down in Extension 37
    Exercise 3: Extension in Lying 38
    Exercise 4: Extension in Standing 40
    Exercise 5: Flexion in Lying 42
    Exercise 6: Flexion in Sitting 44
    Exercise 7: Flexion in Standing 46
    When to Apply the Exercises 47
        When You Have Significant Pain 47
        When to Start Exercising 47
        When Acute Pain Has Subsided 49
        To Prevent Recurrence of Low Back Problems 51
        No Response or Benefit 52
        Recurrence 58

Chapter 6: *When an Episode of Acute Low Back Pain Strikes* 59

Chapter 7: *Special Situations* 61
    Treatment by Repeated End-Range Passive EXercise 61
    Low Back Pain in Pregnancy 62
    Low Back Pain in Athletes 64
    Low Back Pain in the Over 55 66
    Osteoporosis 67

Chapter 8: *Common Remedies* 68
    Medication for Pain Relief 68
    Bed Rest 68
    Acupuncture 68

Chapter 9: *Emergency Back Treatment* 68

Appendix
References 70
The McKenzie Institute International 71

A Chance Discovery

In 1956 in my clinic in Wellington, New Zealand, I observed a remarkable event that has changed the nature of treatment administered worldwide for the alleviation of back pain. This serendipitous event led to the development of the theories and practice that have now become the hallmark of the McKenzie Method of diagnosis and treatment (also known as mechanical diagnosis and therapy or MDT) of common painful back problems.

The chance observation arose from a sudden change in the condition of a patient, Mr. Smith. Mr. Smith had pain to the right of his low back, extending into the buttock and thigh as far as his knee. He had undergone the conventional treatment considered suitable for back pain in that era. After three weeks of heat and ultrasound, his condition had not improved. He had difficulty standing upright. He could bend forward, but when standing could not bend backwards.

I told him to go through to the treatment room and lie face-down on the treatment table, the end of which had been raised for a previous patient. Without adjusting the table, and unnoticed by any of the clinical staff, Mr Smith lay face down with his back arched backward and overstretched for some five minutes. When I returned to commence his treatment, I was extremely concerned to find him lying in what at that time was considered to be a most damaging position. On inquiring as to his welfare, I was astounded to hear him say that this was the best he had been in three weeks. All pain had disappeared from his leg. Furthermore, the pain in the back had moved from the right side to the center. He found he could now bend backward without having severe pain.

When Mr. Smith arose from the treatment table, he could stand upright and he remained improved with no recurrence of leg pain. I placed him in the same position the following day, and this resulted in complete resolution of the remaining symptoms.

The important point is that as Mr. Smith lay in this position, his pain changed location and moved from the leg and right side of his back to the center point just at the waistline. The movement of pain from the leg or buttocks to the middle of the back is now known worldwide as the *centralization phenomenon*.

We now know that when pain moves, as it did in the case of Mr. Smith, the chances of improvement with the methods described in this book are very good. Thanks to the chance observation with Mr. Smith, the McKenzie Method is now provided worldwide by thousands of physiotherapists and doctors treating patients with back pain.

On inquiring as to his welfare, I was astounded to hear him say that this was the best he had been in three weeks. All pain had disappeared from his leg. Furthermore, the pain in the back had moved from the right side to the center. He found he could now bend backward without having severe pain.

My discovery of the centralization phenomenon has provided several important additional benefits. It has enabled physiotherapists who have undergone the McKenzie Institute credentialling or diploma training to acquire the specialist knowledge necessary for implementing the method for the maximum benefit of the patient. While most back pains appear to be similar, in reality the various problems are different and require different solutions. The trained clinician is able to recognize the differences in the spectrum of back pain and provide management for the specific problem.

No other system of diagnosis and treatment has been able to classify these separate entities and provide the necessary management program. Research has shown that physiotherapists holding the McKenzie Institute International credentialling or diploma certificates are best qualified to deliver these methods safely and effectively and obtain the best outcomes for the patient.

treat your own **back**

The Low Back or Lumbar Spine

There are many publications that set out to tell you how to look after your own back and you may well wonder why this one should be any different. The reason is that this book shows you how to put your back 'IN' if you have been unfortunate enough to have put it 'OUT', and in addition it shows you what steps you need to take to avoid a recurrence. I know that you want to get on with the exercises and hasten your recovery process. I know from reports by other patients that they were tempted to skip some of the earlier advice and information and went straight to the exercise section. However, if you too are tempted to skip the early sections, you will miss some of the vital pieces of knowledge that will help cement the base for your complete recovery. *Please read from the beginning!*

Low back pain affects nearly everyone at some stage of active adult life and is one of the most common ailments. It is described as fibrositis, slipped disc, lumbago, arthritis in the back or rheumatism, and when it causes pain extending into the leg, sciatica.

Millions of copies of this book have been sold worldwide. In the twenty-five years since it was first written I have received thousands of letters from grateful patients who have found the solution to their problem. It is probably the most inexpensive treatment you will ever find.

You must be one of the thousands worldwide who continue to have recurring problems with your back. The attacks are not getting less frequent and may be more disabling than previously. Or is it that you have a chronic problem that is not responding to health care clinician, chiropractic or the medication prescribed by your doctor? Or have you had surgery that has failed to correct the problem? You can only be reading this book because all else has so far failed.

Our research tells us that few people buy this book for first-time problems with their back; this book provides the most benefit for people with recurring and chronic problems. Our research also tells us that somewhere between 60% and 75% of the population who have back pain once will experience recurring or chronic back problems. Once taught self-management, most patients willingly take responsibility for their own care. At last there is light at the end of the tunnel!

The majority of over 1000 patients I saw every year for thirty-five years taught me that the only people who really needed my services were those with recurrent or chronic back problems. These patients also taught me that most of them could learn to manage their own problem once they knew what to do. Indeed, it became clear that by applying spinal manipulation or adjustment to all my patients, I was prevented from identifying those who required only exercise. By teaching all patients to perform exercises specifically tailored to suit their own problem, I learned to identify the very few who did require manipulation or adjustment.

The value of *Treat Your Own Back* was measured in a study (Udermann et al.2004) in which the book was given to 62 people with chronic back pain of ten years' average duration. The individuals were then questioned about their back pain nine and eighteen months later. High percentages reported they were still following advice from *Treat Your Own Back* regarding exercises and posture. In these patients, pain magnitude was reduced by over 80% and 75% of them reported no back pain at eighteen months.

To most people, low back pain remains a mystery. It often starts without warning and for no obvious reason. It interferes with simple activities of living, moving about and getting a comfortable night's sleep; and then, just as unexpectedly, the pain subsides. When in acute pain we are usually unable to think clearly about our trouble and simply seek relief from the pain. On the other hand, as soon as we have recovered from an acute episode, most of us quickly forget our low back problems. Once we have developed recurrent low back pain, we cannot do anything else but repeatedly seek assistance to become pain-free. Due to a lack of knowledge and understanding, we are usually unable to deal with present symptoms ourselves and until now have had no way of preventing future low back problems.

Management of your back is *your* responsibility. If you are a typical patient, you have received from many health care professionals a variety of treatments – massage, manipulation, heat, acupuncture, various medications such as anti-inflammatories, and injections. Of course you can get such treatments from specialized physical physiotherapists or health care clinicians, but in the end only *you* can really help yourself. Self-management and treatment of low back pain is now widely accepted; it will be more effective in the long-term management of your low back problems than any other treatment.

The majority of back pains are mechanical in nature; that is, they are caused by problems with the moving parts and therefore certain movements that you make and positions that you adopt can lead to the onset of pain or, if pain is already present, they make it worse. If you are a typical patient, your problem is worse when bending forward for prolonged periods, and especially if sitting for prolonged periods such as when driving. It may be difficult for you to rise from the sitting position and it may take a few minutes before you are able to stand upright properly. Activities such as gardening, digging, vacuuming, making beds or performing any tasks that require you to remain bent or stooped forward for any length of time cause you pain or, if it is already present, make it worse.

If you are like most patients with mechanical back pain, you are better when moving and worse when you remain in one position for prolonged periods. You feel better when walking and when changing your position frequently. You have periods during each day when the pain is much less, and there are times when it is much worse. You may even have periods when you feel no pain at all. Conversely, you may be one who has pain constantly no matter what you do and need to frequently change your position in order to find some relief.

If you have developed low back pain for the first time, you should consult a health care professional such as your family doctor or a specialist clinician who is credentialled or diplomaed by the McKenzie Institute International; to find such a clinician search on the McKenzie Institute International website (www.mckenziemdt.org). Click on your country and then choose 'Locate a Certified McKenzie Therapist'.

Myths About Acute Back Pain

Myth 1: Acute back pain is short-term pain.

The claim that back pain is a short-term problem denies the evidence of research. Many studies show that far from being short-term, over 50% of patients suffer from recurring attacks or have persistent or chronic pain following their initial period of disablement. A study by Croft (1998) in the United Kingdom found that one year following a first attack of acute low back pain, 50% of patients were still complaining of intermittent or persistent symptoms interfering in normal daily activities or work. A study by Enthoven, Skargren, and Oberg (2004) followed patients for five years after their first attack of acute back pain and showed for the first time that large numbers of patients have significant ongoing problems that reduce the quality of their lives and interfere with their livelihoods. This study also found that over 50% of patients had developed long-term problems of recurring and chronic back pain. Another researcher has stated that "back pain is really a lifelong problem for some, and education and explanation to instil self-sufficiency is imperative."

Myth 2: Spinal manipulation is the best and most effective treatment for back pain.

The treatment of back and neck problems by adjustment or manipulation of the spine has in the past been the most popular form of treatment, used mainly by chiropractors and osteopaths. Since the middle of the last century, health care clinician have also adopted this form of treatment. Consequently there are now three professions whose main treatment methods involve the use of spinal manipulation.

Over the past ten to twenty years research has shown that the benefits to be obtained from spinal manipulation have been greatly exaggerated by proponents. The research into manipulation for back pain shows the benefits are unproven because this treatment's effect is minor and often has contradictory results (Koes, 1991, 1996). Because these passive treatments tend to create patient dependence, they are losing credibility. The focus is now on exercise and activity, both of which have the potential to allow patients to manage their own problem and become independent of therapy and clinicians. About 80% of patients with common back problems can be taught the self-manipulation methods outlined in this book. Of those 80%, only 10% will require any form of clinician-applied manipulative therapy.

A study by internationally renowned researchers from the University of Washington in the United States has shown that one month after completing treatment, patients who were taught the McKenzie Method improved to the same degree as patients receiving manipulation by chiropractors. However, the patients receiving the McKenzie Method had fewer treatments to achieve that improvement and 72% of them reported that in the event of recurrence they would manage their own problem. This has great significance for those patients with recurring problems (see Cherkin *et al.* 1998).

It is important that people suffering from back pain are aware that spinal manipulation or adjustive treatments should not be given to the whole population with back pain in order to deliver it to the few who really need it. Spinal manipulation should certainly not be used before self-treatment measures have proven unsuccessful. If you seek treatment from manipulative therapists, chiropractors or osteopaths, it is almost a certainty that you will receive manipulation or adjustment because that is their main weapon for dealing with these problems.

Myth 3: Ultrasound treatment and various electrical therapies are proven to assist recovery from back pain.

Not so! In 1995, the United States Federal Government Agency for Health Care Policy and Research published a list of recommendations to guide those health professionals involved in acute back care. Because there was no supportive scientific evidence, the Agency could not recommend various forms of heat, shortwave diathermy and ultrasound, all of which are commonly used in the treatment of back pain. These treatments provide no long-term benefit and do nothing to treat the underlying problem, nor is there any scientific evidence that they can accelerate healing. Findings such as these have promoted calls for a review of current methods of treatment such as massage, manipulation, ultrasound therapy and other passive treatment modalities. Passive therapies are those in which you lie on a treatment table and the therapist does something to you such as manipulation or ultrasound. Fortunately modern methods are moving away from these treatments as they create patient dependence and are possibly harmful in the long-term, as well as not providing long-term relief.

Myth 4: Back pain is caused by inflammation.

This belief is widespread but generally untrue. While inflammation does occur in the presence of certain conditions such as rheumatoid arthritis and ankylosing spondylitis, sudden onset acute back pain is usually entirely mechanical in nature – that is, it results from the spraining of supporting ligaments around the vertebrae in the low back or distortion that may result from minor displacement of the intervertebral disc. This is commonly referred to as 'slipped disc', but the disc does not actually slip.

Myth 5: Back pain is caused by arthritis or osteoarthritis.

These conditions, which are often described as degeneration of the spine, occur in everyone with ageing. The changes can be seen when the spine is x-rayed. It is actually a process of wearing and repairing, but this does not mean that the wearing is a cause of the pain. X-ray evidence of wearing in the joints of the spine is found in people with back pain as well as in as many of those who have never experienced back pain.

Myth 6: You should take it easy and avoid vigorous activity.

This advice may be necessary for one or two days after the onset of acute pain, but otherwise it is best to regain your mobility as soon as pain permits. The methods described in this book are designed to shorten the recovery process and will, if performed appropriately, reduce your chances of severe recurrence. The secret is to commence the recommended program at the first sign of trouble.

Myth 7: You will have to stop jogging, running, golfing, playing football, tennis etc.

This is untrue and in most cases harmful advice. It is common to mistakenly attribute the onset of back pain to sporting activities. While certainly some back pain can be caused while playing vigorous sport, especially contact sports, there are many other more likely explanations for the onset of the problem. Few back problems are serious enough to justify this advice. While you may have to stop participation in your favourite activity until you recover, permanent abandonment of recreational activity is unnecessary

Myth 8: Back pain is caused by damp conditions or the weather or sitting in a draught.

Climate and the weather have often been accused of causing back and joint pains. There is some as yet invalidated evidence that barometric pressure may have some influence on pain experience during the passage of very high or very low pressure systems, and cold temperatures are also known to increase discomfort in people with inflammatory joint problems. Sitting in a draught has often been blamed for the onset of back pain, but more often it is the sitting posture of the individual that is responsible. None of these events are a cause of joint or back pain.

It has been shown repeatedly that patients require a rational explanation for their problems. They need education in postures and exercises that allow them to remain free of disabling symptoms. They need advice on how to avoid the detrimental forces encountered in daily living and apply beneficial strategies. All of these things are found in this book. Choose your therapist carefully. You should be provided with the information and education you require to manage your own problem. Every patient deserves to have the opportunity to learn how to manage their own back pain and every therapist should be obligated to provide that information.

You should seek advice, particularly if there are complications to your low back pain: for example, when you have constant pain that is referred into your leg all the way to your foot; if you have numbness or weak muscles; especially if you have problems with bladder control and if, in addition to the back pain, you feel unwell. The only health care professionals fully qualified to provide the McKenzie Method are members of the McKenzie Institute International who hold the credentialling certificate or the Diploma in Mechanical Diagnosis & Therapy®. To obtain names of treatment providers trained by the McKenzie Institute, see the directory at the back of this book or use the search feature on the McKenzie Institute International website: www.mckenziemdt.org.

Understanding the Spine

Vertebrae and the Spine

The vertebrae of the human backbone or spine (Photo 1) rest upon one another similarly to a stack of cotton spools (Photo 2).

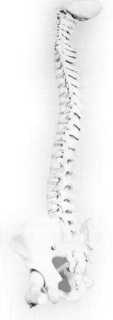

The spine is divided into regions. There are seven vertebrae in the cervical region (neck), twelve vertebrae in the thoracic region (upper back), and five vertebrae in the lumbar region (low back) (Photo 1). Beneath the lumbar vertebrae are found the sacrum and the coccyx (tailbone). It is the low back or lumbar and sacral regions that concern us most in this book.

Each vertebra has a solid part in front, the vertebral body, and a hole in the back (Photo 3). When lined up in the spinal column, these holes form the spinal canal. This canal serves as a protective passageway for the bundle of nerves that extends from head to pelvis – the spinal cord.

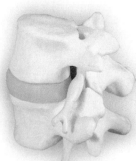

Photo 2) Vertebrae similar to a stack of cotton spools

Special cartilages, called the discs, separate the vertebrae. The discs are located between the vertebral bodies just in front of the spinal cord (Photo 2). Each disc consists of a soft semi-fluid center, the nucleus, which is surrounded and held together by a cartilage ring, called the annulus or annular ligament. The discs are similar to rubber washers and act as shock absorbers. They are able to alter their shape, thus allowing movement of one vertebra on another and of the spine as a whole.

Photo 1) The human spine viewed from side and facing left

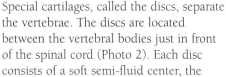

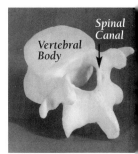

Photo 3) An individual vertabrae

The vertebrae and discs are linked by a series of joints to form the lumbar spine or low back. Each joint is held together by its surrounding soft tissues – that is, a capsule reinforced by ligaments. Ligaments can be likened to the ropes supporting a tent and its poles. If the ropes are subjected to extra strain they are likely to give way and

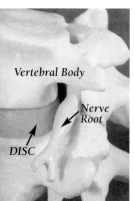

Vertebral Body

Nerve Root

DISC

Photo 4)
Spinal Nerves

the tent will collapse. Every muscle of the back lies over one or more joints of the low back and may extend upwards to the trunk and downwards to the pelvis. At both ends each muscle changes into a tendon by which it attaches itself to different bones. When a muscle contracts, it causes movement in one or more joints.

Between each two vertebrae there is a small opening on either side through which a nerve leaves the spinal canal, the right and left spinal nerves (Photo 4). Amongst other tasks, the spinal nerves supply our muscles with power and our skin with sensation. In other words, it is through the nerves that we can move ourselves and feel temperature, pressure and pain. The nerves are really part of our alarm system: pain is the warning that some structure is about to be damaged or has already sustained damage.

In the lower part of the spine, some of these nerves combine on each side to form the right and left sciatic nerves. These nerves service our legs and when compressed or irritated may cause pain in the leg that often extends below the knee. This is called *sciatica*.

Functions of the Lumbar Spine

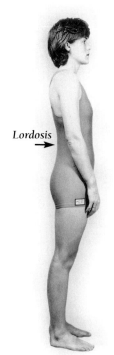

Lordosis
→

Photo 5)
Standing Position

Unlike animals that walk on four feet, in human beings the spine is held in a more or less vertical position, at least during waking and working hours. When we are upright, the lumbar spine bears the compressive weight of the body above it, transmits this weight to the pelvis when sitting and to the feet when standing, walking and running. Thus the lumbar spine, providing a flexible connection between the upper and lower half of the body, protects the spinal cord and also has a greater function in bearing weight. In the evolution of the horizontal-spine posture of animals to the vertical-spine posture of the human, the discs between the vertebrae have adapted to support heavier weights. In addition, the spinal column has developed a series of curves that ingeniously allow for better shock absorption and flexibility.

Natural Posture

The side view of the human body in the standing position (Photo 5) shows that there is an inward curve in the small of the back just above the pelvis. This hollow in the low back is called the *lumbar lordosis*. This is a natural feature of the lumbar spine in all humans, having been formed during the evolutionary process. Our understanding of the function of the lumbar lordosis is an important feature of this book.

When standing upright the lordosis is naturally present, although it varies from person to person. The lordosis is lost whenever the low back is rounded as occurs during sitting and bending forward. If the lordosis is lost often and for long enough periods, then low back problems may develop. The ligaments become fatigued or overstretched and may give way, resulting in another painful back episode.

Mechanical Pain

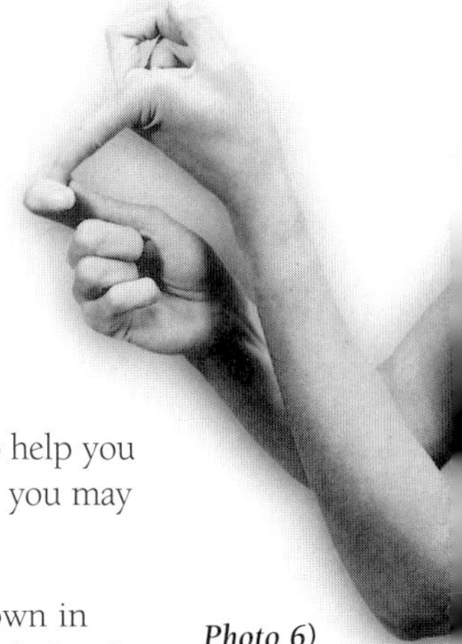

Pain of mechanical origin occurs when the joint between two bones has been placed in a position that overstretches the surrounding ligaments and other soft tissues. This is true for mechanical pain in any joint of the body, including the spine. To help you understand how easily some mechanical pains can be produced, you may like to try a simple experiment.

First, bend one finger backward until you feel a strain, as shown in Photo 6. If you keep your finger in this position, you initially feel only minor discomfort, but as time passes, pain eventually develops. In some cases, pain caused by prolonged stretching may take as much as an hour to appear.

Photo 6)
Bend the finger
until you feel
the strain

Try the experiment once more, but now keep bending the finger past the point of strain until you feel the immediate sensation of pain. You have overstretched, and your pain warning system is telling you that to continue movement in that particular direction will cause damage.

The pain warning tells you to stop overstretching to avoid damage and when you do so, the pain ceases immediately. No damage has occurred and the pain has gone. No lasting problems arise from this short-lived strain providing you take note of the pain warning system.

If you fail to heed the warning and keep the finger in the overstretched position, the ligaments and surrounding soft tissues that hold the joint together will eventually tear. This tearing will result in an ache that continues even when you stop overstretching. The pain reduces in intensity but continues even when the finger is at rest. The pain increases with movement performed in the wrong direction and will not cease until some healing has occurred. Healing may take several days, but would be prolonged if every day you were to continue to apply the same strains to the finger. *The same things happen when you overstretch the ligaments in your back.*

Mechanical Low Back Pain

If an engineer were to examine which area in the back is subjected mostly to mechanical stress, he would conclude that most strain must be placed on that part of the spine that is located just above its junction with the pelvis. This conclusion is correct, for statistics show that back problems arise more often in the low back than in any other part of the spine.

Just as pain arises in the overstretched finger as I have described above, pain can also arise in the low back from prolonged overstretching of the ligaments in this area. Pain produced by overstretching in this manner is common and arises particularly when we develop poor postural habits. Whenever we remain in a relaxed position, whether standing, sitting or lying, prolonged overstretching can easily occur.

When pain arises because we have allowed our posture to slouch, it is really our own fault. This type of strain is easily avoided and once we have been properly educated, the prevention of pain produced in this manner becomes our responsibility. Pain arising from prolonged stretching is called the *Postural Syndrome*.

However, mechanical pain may also be caused by overstretching of such severity that some tissues are actually damaged. Damage from overstretching may occur when an outside force places an excessive strain on the low back. For example, this type of strain can occur due to a fall or from a contact sport such as football when players are tackled. Lifting excessive weights is also likely to cause overstretching and damage to the supporting ligaments of the spinal joints. These types of injury cannot easily be avoided as they occur unexpectedly.

When soft tissues surrounding a joint are overstretched, it is usually the ligaments that first feel pain. When the spinal joints are considered there are additional factors, for the surrounding ligaments are also the retaining walls for the soft discs that act as shock absorbers between the vertebrae. Overstretching of these will, under certain circumstances, affect the discs. This may significantly influence the intensity of your pain, the distribution of your pain and its behaviour, which may be made better or worse by certain movements or positions.

Complications of another sort arise when the ligament surrounding the disc is injured to such an extent that the disc loses its ability to absorb shock and its outer wall becomes weakened. This allows the soft inside of the disc to bulge outwards and, in extreme cases, to burst through the outer ligament, causing severe pain. When the disc bulges far enough it may press painfully on the sciatic nerve. This can cause pain or other symptoms (numbness, sensation of pins and needles, weakness) that may be felt well away from the source of the trouble, for example in the lower leg or foot.

Should the soft inside of the disc bulge excessively, the disc may become severely distorted. This causes the vertebrae to tilt forward or to one side and prevents it from lining up properly during movement. In this case some movements are blocked partially or completely and any movement may cause severe pain. This is why some people with severe back pain are forced to stand with the trunk off-center or bent forward. Those experiencing a sudden onset of pain and the inability to straighten up or move the back properly are likely to have some bulging of the soft disc material. This need not be a cause for alarm. The exercises described in this book are carefully designed to reduce any disturbance of this nature. Pain from distortion or displacement of the disc is called the *Derangement Syndrome*.

This problem can be explained better by trying this experiment. First, wet both hands and place a cake of soap in the middle of your palm. Then press the heels of your hands together. The soap moves away from the point of highest pressure and is displaced from between your fingers. You can avoid the displacement by quickly reversing the point of pressure so that the soap comes back to the center of your palms.

The disc between the vertebrae behaves in a similar manner. If you bend forward briefly, there is an adjustment in location of the soft center of the disc that is displaced slightly backward. As you come upright, that slight displacement is reversed and corrected. However, if you bend forward for prolonged periods, the backward displacement can become excessive and may cause pain, but the soft disc cannot usually escape and is retained by the strong ligaments. As long as the ligaments are intact, you can prevent significant displacement by standing upright and bending backward. This reverses the distortion and any displacement and the pain subsides. Under certain circumstances, if the supporting ligaments are weakened sufficiently, the displacement of the soft disc can cause pressure on the sciatic nerve and cause pain in the buttock and/or the leg. It is still possible to reverse this displacement, but you must be more careful when it comes to the application of the exercises. Since this book was first published research conducted in the United States and United Kingdom has proven that the disc between the vertebrae moves as I first described it in 1980, although that idea was strenuously challenged by the established medical wisdom of the day.

In 1983, at an American Orthopaedic Association meeting, I was asked to address one prominent orthopaedic surgeon of the day stood and challenged me saying, "Mr McKenzie, we orthopaedic surgeons have been in there [meaning at surgery] and the disc does not move. You must not keep on saying that!" [Twenty-five years later he apologized to me for his error.]

Once soft tissues are damaged, pain is felt until healing is complete and function is fully restored. It is important that during the healing process you avoid movements that pull the healing surfaces apart. For instance, if you have overstretched ligaments of the low back by bending forward, it is likely that any repetition of this movement will continue to open and separate the healing tissues and this will further delay repair. If, however, you avoid bending forward and instead keep a hollow in the low back, the damaged surfaces remain together and healing is not interrupted.

It is perhaps difficult to visualize this occurring in the low back. Imagine that you have accidentally cut across the back of your knuckle. If you were to bend the injured finger joint every day, you would open up the wound and delay recovery. However, by keeping the finger straight for about a week, you would allow the healing surfaces to remain together and complete healing would result. You could then bend the finger without risking any further damage. The same strategy works for the problems arising in the low back.

When tissues heal they form scar tissue. Scar tissue is less elastic than normal tissue and tends to shorten over time. If shortening occurs, movement may stretch the scars and produce pain in the same area in which it first appeared. This can create the impression that you are still injured whereas in reality healing is complete and you are pulling on the scar itself. Unless appropriate exercises are performed to restore normal flexibility, the healed tissue may produce a continuous source of back pain and/or stiffness for years. Even though the original damage is repaired, the scar itself restricts movement and causes pain when stretched. Pain caused by stretching scar tissue is called the *Dysfunction Syndrome*.

Pain Location

The location of pain caused by low back problems varies from one person to another. In a first attack pain is usually felt in the center of the back, at or near the belt line or just to one side, and in general it subsides within a few days. (Figure 1) In subsequent attacks pain may extend to the buttock, and later still to the back or outside of the thigh, down to the knee (Figure 2) or below the knee down to the ankle or foot. Less often pain is felt in the front of the thigh to the knee. Pain may vary with movement or with position; the intensity of the pain can change, or the location of the pain can alter – for example, one movement may cause buttock pain, and another may cause the pain to leave the buttock and appear in the low back.

If you have a severe problem, in addition to low back pain you may experience significant numbness or muscular weakness in the lower leg.

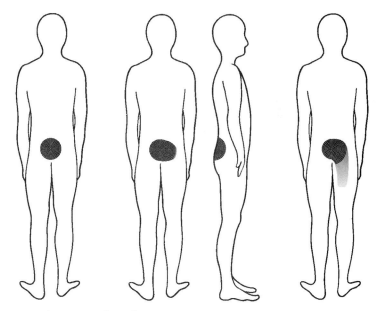

Figure 1) First incident of pain

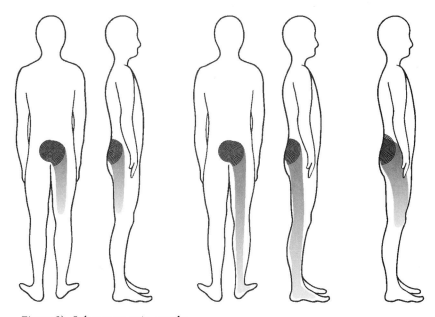

Figure 2) Subsequent pain attacks

Self-Treatment

Most people will benefit from the advice given in this book, and many will completely rid themselves of pain. Only a few patients – perhaps 10 or 15% – will fail to derive any benefit or favorable response. Lasting improvement can only be obtained if you are conscientious with both the exercises and especially posture correction. You can commence the exercise program immediately, provided you follow the various precautions described later.

When Self-Treatment Does Not Work

Once you have started the exercises, carefully watch your pain pattern. If your pain was steadily worsening before you started this program and does not begin to subside after the first two weeks, or if your symptoms consistently increase immediately following the exercises and you remain worse over the following two days, you should discontinue the exercises and seek advice from your McKenzie Institute credentialled or diplomaed health care clinician.

Diagnosing Your Problem

To assist you in diagnosing your problem, the following section is *essential* for your complete understanding of back pain. *You should not commence the exercise programme in any of the following situations:*

- if you have severe pain in the leg below the knee and experience sensations of weakness, numbness or pins and needles in the foot and toes

- if you have developed low back problems following a recent severe accident

- if following a recent severe episode of low back pain, you have developed bladder problems

- if you are feeling generally unwell in conjunction with this attack of low back pain

- if you have a previous history of cancer or tumor

- if you develop a fever, high temperature, or start sweating

- if you develop any other symptoms in addition to your back pain.

If you still have any doubts after completing the checklist, you must seek advice from your family doctor

To help you to determine whether you can treat your low back pain successfully without further assistance, you should answer the following checklist:

- Are there periods in the day when you have no pain? Even ten minutes? . . . . Yes / No

- Is the pain confined to areas above the knee? . . . . Yes / No

- Are you generally worse when sitting for prolonged periods or on rising from the sitting position? . . . . Yes / No

- Are you generally worse during or right after prolonged bending or stooping as in bed-making, vacuuming, ironing, concreting, digging or gardening? . . . . Yes / No

- Are you generally worse when getting up in the morning, but improve after about half an hour? . . . . Yes / No

- Are you generally worse when inactive and better when on the move? . . . . Yes / No

- Are you generally better when walking? . . . . Yes / No

- Are you generally better when lying face down? When testing this you may feel worse for the first few minutes after which time the pain subsides; in this case the answer to the question is 'yes'. . . . . Yes / No

- Have you had several episodes of low back pain over the past months or years? . . . . Yes / No

- Between episodes, are you able to move fully in all directions without pain? . . . . Yes / No

- Between episodes, are you pain-free?. . . . . Yes / No

- If you have pain in the buttocks, or the upper or lower leg, does it sometimes stop completely, even though you may still have pain in the back?. . . . . Yes / No

If you have answered 'yes' to all the questions, you are an ideal candidate for the self-treatment programme outlined in this book.

If you have answered 'yes' to five or more questions, your chances to benefit from self-treatment are good and you should commence the program.

If you have answered 'yes' to only four or fewer questions, then some form of specialized treatment may be required and you should consult the directory included at the back of this book for a therapist credentialled or diplomaed by the McKenzie Institute International.

Common Causes of Low Back Pain

Consequences of Postural Neglect

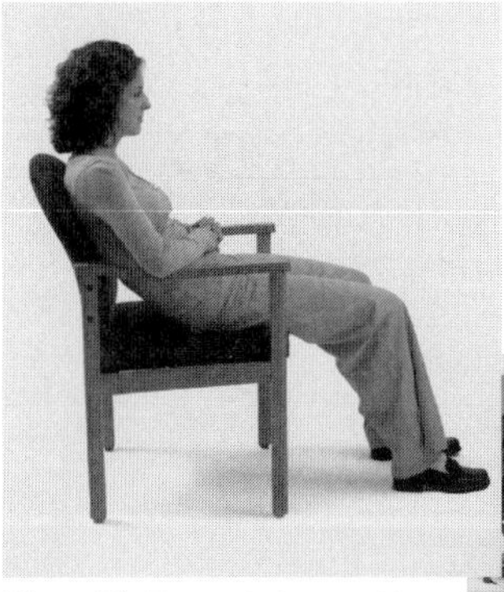

Photo 7) Poor sitting position

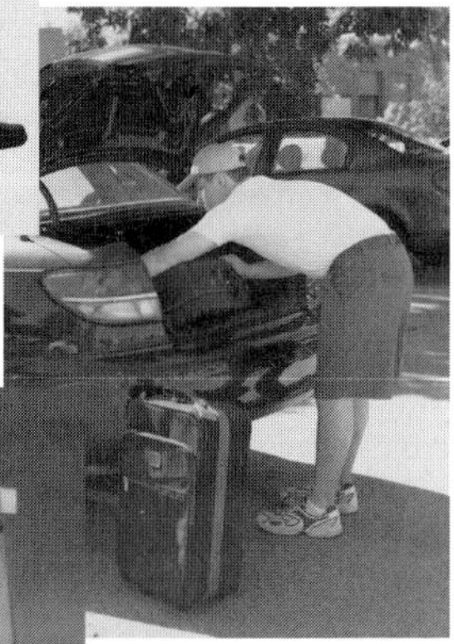

The most common cause of low back pain is postural stress. This type of low back pain is frequently brought on by sitting for a long time in a poor position (Photo 7), poor lifting technique (Photo 8), prolonged forward bending in bad working positions (Photo 9) or standing and lying for a long time in a poor position (Photo 10). When you look carefully at these photos, you will see that the low back is rounded and the lordosis has disappeared.

Photo 8) Poor lifting technique

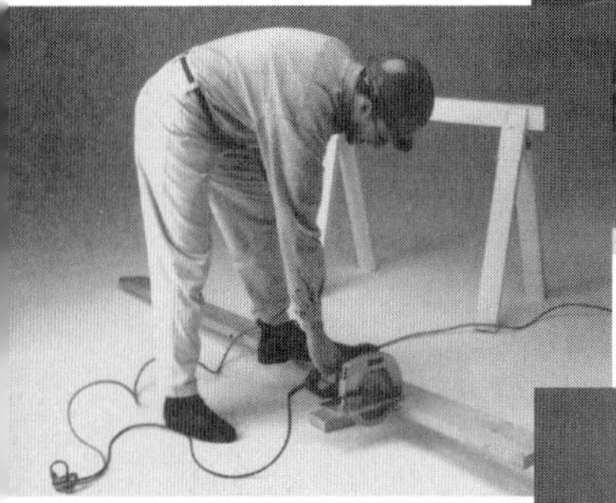

Photo 9) Awkward bending position

Unfortunately many of us spend much of our work and leisure time with the low back in a flexed rounded position and lose the lordosis completely. On the other hand we seldom or never increase it to its maximum. If you reduce the lordosis for long periods at a time and never properly restore it, you eventually lose the ability to form the hollow. It is known that a flattened low back is frequently associated with chronic low back problems.

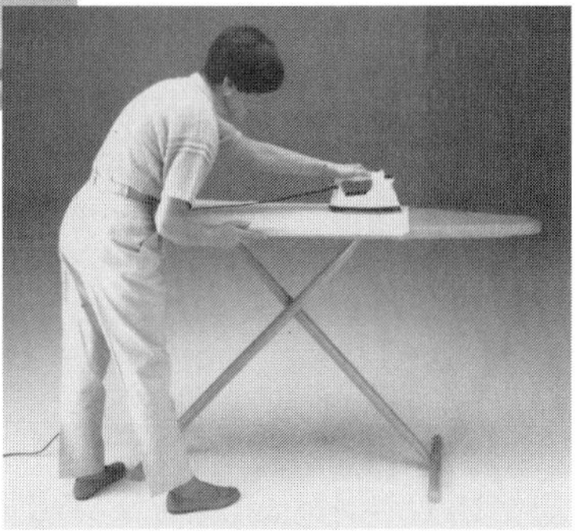

Photo 10) Poor standing position

Some people who habitually adopt poor postures and remain unaware of the underlying cause experience back pain throughout their lifetimes simply because they were not in possession of the necessary information to correct the postural faults.

When pains of postural origin are first felt they are easily eliminated merely by correcting one's posture. As time passes, however, if uncorrected the habitual poor posture causes changes to the structure and shape of the joints; excessive wear occurs, with loss of elasticity resulting in premature ageing of the joints. The effects of poor posture in the long term, therefore, can be just as severe and harmful as the effects of injury.

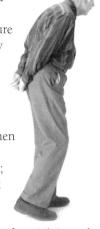

Deformities in the elderly are the visible effects of poor postural habit. There are secondary and sometimes severe consequences when these effects are transmitted to our body organs: the lungs are constricted and our breathing is affected as the back becomes bent; the stomach and other internal organs are deprived of their correct support and may well be affected adversely.

The bent, stooped posture considered by many to be one of the inevitable consequences of aging (Photo 11) is not at all inevitable and the time to commence preventive action is now. If you stand fully erect and bend fully backward once a day, you need never lose the ability to perform that action and therefore need never become bent, stooped and impaired in so many ways.

Photo 11) Stooped posture in ageing

Sitting

A poor sitting posture commonly produces low back pain. Once low back problems have developed, a poor sitting posture perpetuates or worsens those problems. Most people sitting for prolonged periods eventually adopt a slouched posture. When next you go to a restaurant or to the movies look at the posture of those around you. You will see that most people have allowed their backs to slouch and become rounded. Poor posture is extremely widespread in our communities and is due partially to our increasingly sedentary lifestyles.

When we sit in a certain position for a few minutes, the muscles that support our low back become tired and relax. Our body sags and this results in the slouched sitting posture (Photo 12). If we maintain a slouched sitting posture for long enough, it causes overstretching of ligaments and pain. Once the slouched sitting posture has become a habit and is maintained most of the time, it may also cause distortion of the discs contained in the vertebral joints. Once this occurs, movements as well as positions produce pain.

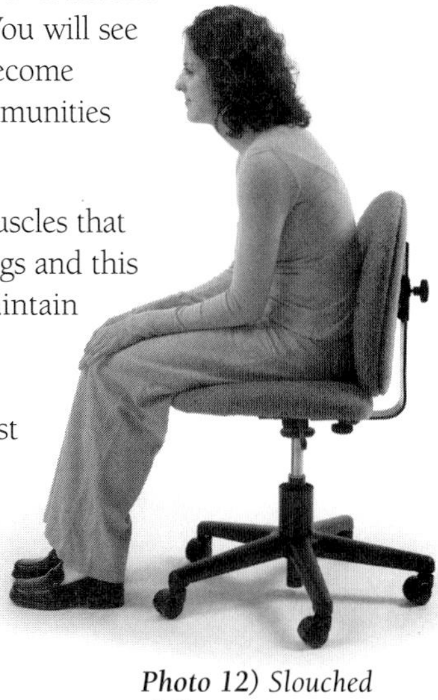

Photo 12) Slouched sitting posture

Prolonged Sitting

It follows that people with sedentary office jobs easily develop low back problems as they often sit with a rounded back for hours (Photo 13). If you are a sedentary worker, you may go through the following stages of gradually increasing back problems unless you take steps to rectify the cause.

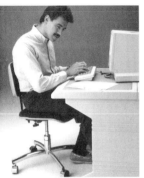

At first you may only experience discomfort in the low back *while* sitting for a prolonged period of time or on attempting to arise from sitting. In this case the pain is caused by slight overstretching of soft tissues, and it takes a few seconds for these tissues to recover. The pain at this stage is short-lived. Later you find that on attempting to stand you have increased pain and must walk carefully for a short distance before you can straighten up fully. The pain may even persist after you have gained the upright posture. It is likely that some minor distortion has occurred in one of the lumbar joints which may need a few minutes to recover.

Photo 13) Sitting for prolonged periods with a rounded back leads to low back problems

Eventually you may reach the stage when you experience acute or agonizing pain on standing and are unable to straighten up at all. In this case there is major distortion in the affected joint, which cannot regain its normal shape quickly enough to allow pain-free movement. Whenever a movement is attempted, the disc bulge increases the strain on the already overstretched surrounding tissues. In addition, the disc bulge may pinch the sciatic nerve, leading to pain and other symptoms in the leg.

Posture and Sitting

Sitting Correctly for Prolonged Periods

Of these postural stresses, the poor sitting posture is by far the one most commonly at fault. To avoid the development of low back pain due to prolonged poor sitting, (Photo 14) it is necessary to sit correctly (Photo 15) and to interrupt prolonged sitting at regular intervals. If at the present time you have pain resulting from factors other than just poor posture, special exercises may need to be performed in addition to the postural correction. This section describes only the exercises required to reduce postural stresses and obtain postural correction. The self-treatment exercises for relief of pain and increase of function are dealt with in the next chapter.

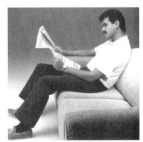

Photo 14) Poor sitting posture

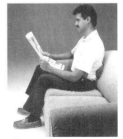

Photo 15) Correct sitting posture

Correction of the Sitting Posture

You may have had the habit for many years of sitting slouched without low back pain, but once low back problems have developed you must no longer sit in the old way. From now on you must pay attention to your sitting posture.

In order to sit correctly you must first learn how to form a lordosis in the low back while sitting. Therefore you must become fully practiced in what I have called the slouch–overcorrect procedure. Once you have achieved this, you must learn how to maintain a lordosis in the low back while sitting for prolonged periods.

How to Form a Lordosis Using the Slouch-Overcorrect Procedure

You must restore the lordosis slowly and with caution, never quickly or with jerky movements. You must allow some time for the distorted joint to regain its normal shape and position: a sudden or violent movement may retard this process, increase the strain in and around the affected joint, and thus result in an increase of low back pain.

Sit on a stool of chair height or sideways on a kitchen or dining chair. Allow yourself to slouch completely (Photo 16). Now you are ready to commence the **slouch–overcorrect** procedure:

- relax for a few seconds in the slouched position, then draw yourself up and accentuate the lordosis as far as possible (Photo 17). This is the extreme of the correct sitting position

- hold yourself in this position for a few seconds, then return to the fully relaxed position

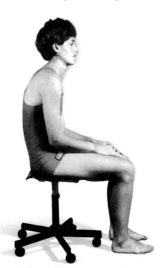

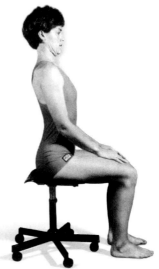

Photo 16) Extreme of relaxed slouched position

Photo 17) Extreme of good position

The movement from the slouched to the upright sitting position should be done in such a way that you move rhythmically from the extreme of the bad to the extreme of the good sitting posture. The exercise must be performed ten to fifteen times per session and the sessions are to be repeated three times per day, preferably morning, noon and evening. You should also perform this exercise whenever pain arises as a result of sitting poorly. Each time you repeat this movement cycle you must make sure that the movement is performed to the maximum possible degree, especially towards the extreme of the good position.

Maintenance of the Lordosis

You have just learned how to find the extreme of the good sitting posture. It is not possible to sit in this way for long periods as it is a position of considerable strain, and if maintained for excessive periods could actually cause pain. To sit comfortably and correctly you must sit just short of the extreme good posture. To find this position you

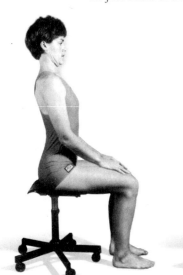
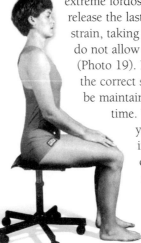

must first sit with your low back in extreme lordosis (Photo 18) and then release the last 10% of the lordosis strain, taking care to ensure that you do not allow the low back to flatten (Photo 19). Now you have reached the correct sitting posture, which can be maintained for any length of time. When sitting like this you maintain the lordosis in the low back with your own muscular effort; it requires constant attention and constant effort and you cannot fully relax. Whenever you sit in a seat without a backrest, you must sit in this way.

Photo 18) Extreme of good position

Photo 19) Correct sitting position

The Lumbar Roll

As few seats or chairs provide adequate support for the lower back, I found it necessary to provide my patients with a portable lumbar roll that could be used in the car, lounge seat and at the dining table. When I realized that a support was vital for my patients if they were to remain pain-free I found that no one knew of anything suitable to purchase. Therefore, in the early days before the Original McKenzie® range of rolls (Photos 20 and 21) went into commercial production, my wife made them herself, on our kitchen table. Now I believe there are hundreds of other companies worldwide manufacturing lumbar rolls for back support.

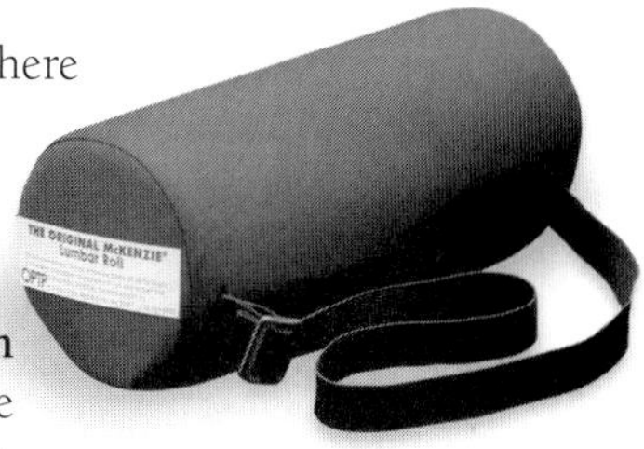

A portable lumbar roll is essential equipment for people with ongoing back problems. When sitting on a seat **with a back-rest** (supported sitting) a lumbar roll will facilitate the maintenance of a correct lordosis and posture.

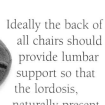

Photo 20) The Original McKenzie® Lumbar Roll

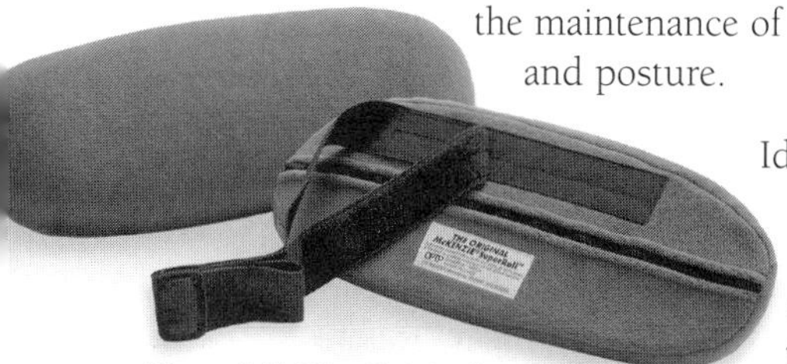

Photo 21) The Original McKenzie® SuperRoll™

Ideally the back of all chairs should provide lumbar support so that the lordosis, naturally present during standing, is also maintained while sitting (Photo 22). It is relatively easy in most countries these days, to find seating that has some degree of lumbar support but few seats or chairs provide adequate support for the low back (Photo 23) and it is usually still necessary to use a lumbar roll. You can purchase an Original McKenzie® lumbar roll specifically designed for the purpose, from the licensed supplier nearest you, listed at the back of this book. Proceeds from the sale of the Original McKenzie® spinal supports have been, and continue to be, donated for research of improved methods of treatment for musculoskeletal disorders and to provide relevant education for clinicians. A regular cushion or small rolled up towel should not be relied upon for long-term use, but may be of some assistance in an emergency.

On one occasion, when flying from New York to Zurich, I noticed that a fellow passenger was using an Original McKenzie® Lumbar Roll. I introduced myself and enquired how he came to have one of my inventions. He said that his doctor in Zurich "prescribed McKenzie Lumbar Rolls for all his patients", and added that he "never leaves home without it."

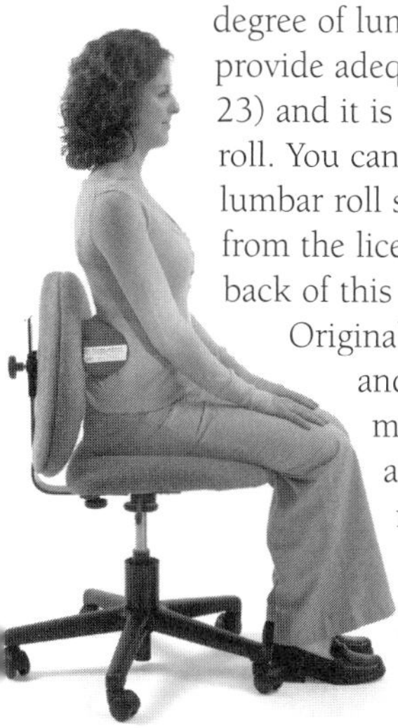

Photo 22) A lumbar roll helps you maintain correct lordosis and posture

The aim is first to restore the correct posture and then to maintain it. It may take up to a week of practice to master this fully. As a rule, pain of postural origin will decrease as your sitting posture improves and you will have no pain once you maintain the correct posture. The pain will readily recur in the first few weeks should you allow yourself to slouch while sitting. Eventually you will remain completely pain-free even when you forget your posture; however, never again should you allow yourself to sit slouched for long periods.

When first starting these procedures or the exercises to correct your sitting posture, you will experience some new pains that are different from your original pain and may be felt in other places.

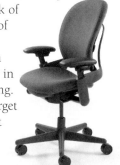

Photo 23) A well designed desk chair

New pains are the result of performing new exercises and maintaining new positions. They should be expected and will wear off in a few days, provided postural correction is continued on a regular basis. I always suspect that if the patient does not complain of new pains, they have not been doing the exercises correctly or frequently enough.

The McKenzie Institute International commissioned a study to examine the effects of sitting with, and without, a lumbar roll. Patients in the group using the lumbar roll were required to use it at home, at the office and when driving. The results showed conclusively that those patients using a portable lumbar roll when sitting experienced much less or even no pain compared to those not using a lumbar support (see Williams *et al.* 1991).

Regular Interruption of Prolonged Sitting

Travelling for long distances without regular breaks that permit you to restore lordosis may cause a gradual and progressive attack of low back pain or may aggravate existing problems. Nearly everyone will be aware of some stiffness or discomfort in the low back after a few hours in a car without interruption. If you already have back problems, such a journey may be risky for you.

In order to minimize the risks associated with prolonged sitting, it is necessary that you use a lumbar roll and (Photo 24) interrupt sitting at regular intervals and before pain starts. For example, when undertaking long car journeys, you should stop the car every hour, get

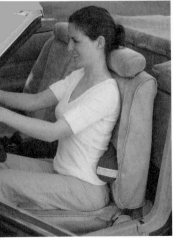

out and bend backward five or six times (see Exercise 4, in chapter 5) and walk for a few minutes. This reduces the pressure within the discs and relieves the stresses on the surrounding tissues. As most airlines continue to provide seating that can damage the human spine, you should, when flying long distances, use an Original McKenzie® AirBack inflatable lumbar roll (Photo 25) and regularly stand and walk up and down the aisle of the plane. This is not only important for the sake of your back, but is also necessary to assist in the stimulation of the circulation in the legs. These are simple measures you can take that significantly reduce the risk of another episode of back pain.

Photo 24) Use a lumbar roll when driving, particularly on long journeys

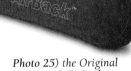

Photo 25) the Original McKenzie® AirBack inflatable lumbar roll

Standing

When we are standing the lordosis is naturally present, but in some individuals, when the standing posture is maintained for a long time, the lordosis can become excessive and pain produced is of a different nature than that occurring during prolonged bending.

Poor standing postures (Photo 26) and poor lying postures are frequent causes of back pain. You may have already found that your back pain appears only if you stand for long periods or only after you get into bed. Pain that behaves in this way is frequently caused by poor posture alone. If this is the case, it is easily rectified.

In the summer of 1965 I took my wife and children on a five-hour road trip to Lake Taupo, a holiday resort in the center of the North Island of New Zealand. In those days the McKenzie Method was pretty much known only to me. During the journey, in the distance on the side of the road, I could see a parked car. Once alongside the car I could see a man lying face down doing half push-ups. I thought this can only be a patient of mine so I stopped the car and asked him how he was? He looked up, and recognizing me, said simply "just doing my exercises as instructed". I replied, "Just checking". That was all that was said and I went on my way. Patients do follow instructions if they understand why they have been given them and they derive benefit from them.

Prolonged Standing

Some people always get low back pain when standing in one place for a long time. Just as muscles tire and relax when we sit for long periods, they also do when we stand for long periods, allowing us to slouch. When we stand relaxed, however, the lordosis becomes excessive and the low back hangs in an extreme position. If your low back pain is produced during prolonged standing, you can find relief by correcting your standing posture.

Correction of the Standing Posture

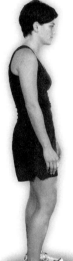

Photo 26) Poor standing posture

To stand correctly, you must hold your low back in a position of reduced lordosis. To find this position, first stand relaxed. Allow the chest to sag and the abdomen to protrude slightly; this places the lower lumbar joints in an extreme lordosis. Now reduce the lordosis by standing as tall as you can. Lift the chest up, pull in your stomach muscles, and tighten your buttocks (Photo 27). You have now reached the correct standing posture. In this standing position you reduce the lordosis with your own muscular effort. To begin with it is difficult to effectively hold this position, but with practice this new position can be held for long periods without discomfort.

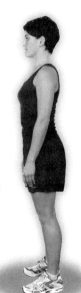

Photo 27) Correction of the standing posture

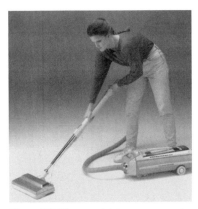

Photo 28) *Many activities cause you to bend forward*

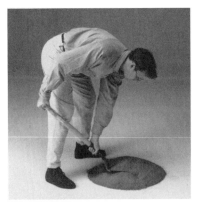

Photo 29) *Working in prolonged stooped positions*

Working in Stooped Positions

When standing with your back straight, the stresses on discs and ligaments in your low back are considerably lower than when you stand with your back bent forward. Many activities around the home may cause you to bend – for example; gardening, sweeping, digging, vacuuming, making the bed, etc. (Photo 28). Occupations requiring prolonged stooped postures are abundant: assembly line workers, bricklayers, electricians, plumbers, carpenters, cleaners, gardeners, nurses, mechanics, etc. All are required to bend forward for prolonged periods every day (Photo 29). While working in these bent positions, you are more likely to sustain back problems in the first four or five hours of the day. I made this discovery simply by recording times of onset of pain in thousands of patients. Although I reported this evidence in 1979 it was not until 1998 that a researcher named Stover Snook in the United States published his study findings confirming the risk. He reported that "Patients with chronic low back pain were found to experience significant improvements in pain and disability by reducing bending forward activities early in the morning".

In order to minimize the risks involved in prolonged forward bending, the stooped position should be interrupted at regular intervals before pain starts. Stand upright and bend backward five or six times (see Exercise 4). When this is done before pain starts, it usually prevents the development of significant low back pain; and remember, because the discs in your spine swell up naturally during your non-weight-bearing hours, you are especially at risk in the first half of your day, so make sure you always do everything correctly during this period.

LIFTING

Lifting objects with your back rounded (Photo 30) has been found to raise the pressure in the discs to a much higher level than that existing when the weight is held with the body upright and the lordosis present. Just as back problems associated with bending seem to occur frequently in the first four or five hours of the day, so it is with lifting, especially if you are lifting repeatedly and frequently. If you use an incorrect lifting technique while lifting heavier objects, you may cause damage and, of course, sudden severe pain.

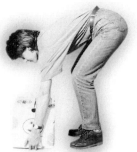

Photo 30) Poor lifting technique

In order to minimise the risks involved in lifting, always use the correct lifting technique (Photos 31a-e).

Correct Lifting Technique

Throughout lifting you must attempt to retain the hollow in your low back (Photos 31). The lift should be applied by straightening the legs. Avoid using the back as a crane to lift the weight. Correct lifting technique involves the following:

- stand close to the load, have firm footing and a wide stance
- accentuate the lordosis
- bend your knees to go down to the load and keep your back straight
- get a secure grip and hold the load as close to you as possible
- lean back to stay in balance and lift the load by straightening the knees
- lift steadily; do not jerk
- when upright, shift your feet to turn and avoid twisting the low back
- The same technique should be used in reverse when lowering the heavy load.

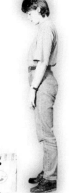 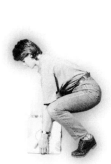 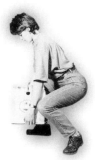 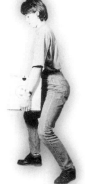 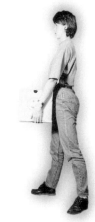

Photo 31a   *Photo 31b*   *Photo 31c*   *Photo 31d*   *Photo 31e*

Stand upright and bend backward five or six times immediately before and after lifting (Photo 32), especially when a single heavy lift is involved. If there are many objects to be lifted, you should frequently interrupt the lifting and repeat the backward bending exercise. This is particularly important if you have been in a stooped position or have been sitting for a prolonged period immediately before you start lifting.

For example, many truck drivers after driving for prolonged periods are then called upon to remove heavy loads. Removing heavy suitcases from the trunk of the car immediately after a long ride is another example of this high risk situation (Photo 33). By standing upright and bending backward a few times before and after lifting, you correct any distortion that may have developed and reduce the likelihood of another attack of acute pain.

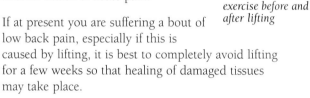

Photo 32) Extension exercise before and after lifting

If at present you are suffering a bout of low back pain, especially if this is caused by lifting, it is best to completely avoid lifting for a few weeks so that healing of damaged tissues may take place.

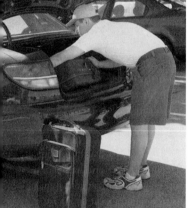

Photo 33) Incorrect lifting techniques after a long car ride are particularly risky

RELAXING AFTER VIGOROUS ACTIVITY

Over the years I have heard many people complain that they develop back pains after engaging in vigorous sport and heavy activities such as jogging, tennis or gardening. However, often after activity we sit and relax, very often collapsing slouched in a chair. Once we feel the onset of pain, we automatically project blame to the activity that we have just completed. We should instead consider that the pain has resulted from the posture we have since adopted.

Over the years I have advised many athletes, including three of the world's top golfers. My question to each was, "Do you have pain while participating or does the pain commence only after you have finished?" Many of those athletes and two of the golfers replied that they felt nothing during the activity, but the pain always commenced later. When asked to be more specific, the typical response was that "the pain commenced while relaxing later." My question then was, "What sort of relaxing?" The reply was always: "Sitting!" (Photo 34) The answer to the problem is that after vigorous activity, you must sit correctly with a back roll or support. Thoroughly exercised joints of the spine distort easily if they are subsequently placed in a slouched position for long periods.

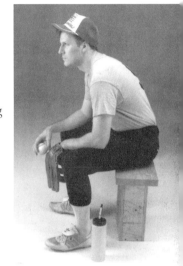

Photo 34) Slouched sitting after activity can promote pain

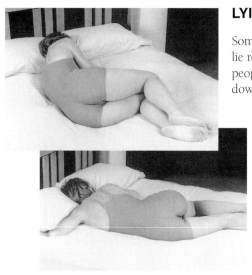

Photo 35) Common sleeping positions

LYING AND RESTING

Some people have low back pain when they lie resting in certain positions, and a few people have low back pain *only* when they lie down.

If you have low back pain only when lying down, or if you regularly wake in the morning with a stiff and painful low back that was not painful the night before, there is likely to be something wrong with the surface on which you are lying or the position in which you sleep (Photos 35). It is a comparatively easy task to correct the surface on which you are lying, but rather difficult to influence the position you adopt while sleeping. Once you are asleep, you may regularly change your position or toss and turn. Unless a certain position causes so much discomfort that it wakes you, you have no real idea of the various positions you assume while sleeping.

Many people with back problems are told never to lie face down when in bed. There is no evidence whatsoever to suggest that this is harmful to the back. On the contrary, it may well be that your back ceases to be painful in the face-down position. If you have not already discovered the effects of lying face down, you should experiment to see what effect this has on your problem the next time you experience pain while lying. Certainly there are some low back problems that are aggravated by lying in this way. If you have severe sciatica, lying face down is nearly always impossible.

Correction of Surface

There are two simple ways in which you may be able to reduce strains on your low back caused by a faulty lying position. The first and most important way is to lie with a supportive lumbar roll around your waist. The roll supports your low back as you rest and prevents strain that can develop when you lie on your side or back.

Photo 36) the Original McKenzie® night roll

The Original McKenzie® night Roll has been specifically designed for the purpose and is available from the resources listed at the back of this book. The night Roll comes in different lengths so you will need to let the supplier know your waist measurement. The night Roll is long enough to support you when lying on your back or on either side. Wrap the roll around your waist and tie it in front to ensure that it remains in place where you normally wear your belt; otherwise, should the roll move up or down during your sleep, it may actually increase your night pain. To get the best 'fit' you should hold the roll in place around your waist, lie down on your bed and then tie it snugly in front. You may need to move it slightly up or down to get it in the right place. Generally, when you lie on your side the roll should fill the natural hollow in the body contour between pelvis and rib cage, and when you lie on your back,

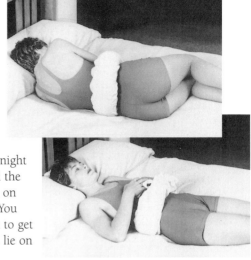

Photo 37) Correction of sleeping surface and posture with a night roll

the roll should support the low back in moderate lordosis (Photo 37). Sleeping with a night Roll may initially be uncomfortable but this should pass within a few days.

The second way is to ensure that your mattress does not sag. The mattress itself should not be too hard; in fact, a soft mattress can be extremely comfortable provided it is placed on a firm support. A study reported that patients who slept on the medium-firm mattresses were more likely to report reduced back pain in bed, reduced back pain upon rising from the bed, and less back pain related to disability than the patients who slept on a firm mattress (Kovacs *et al.* 2003).

If you have tried these suggestions without benefit, you should consult a clinician credentialled or diplomaed by the McKenzie Institute International.

COUGHING AND SNEEZING

Coughing and sneezing while you are bent forward or sitting may cause a sudden attack of low back pain or aggravate existing back pain. If you sense the need to cough or sneeze, you should try to stand upright and bend backward so that your low back is hollow at the moment you cough or sneeze. Should you not be able to stand up, then you must at least lean backward and make the best possible lordosis.

Understanding the McKenzie Method

YOUR UNDERSTANDING OF THIS CHAPTER IS ESSENTIAL
FOR SUCCESSFUL SELF-TREATMENT.

Aim of the Exercises

**The exercises described in this book are not designed to
strengthen the muscles of your back.** They are designed to effect
changes in the internal components in and around the joints of the
spine. In doing so, you will notice that there are simultaneous changes
in the location or the intensity levels of your pain. **The manner in
which these changes occur allow you to diagnose your problem.**

These specific responses show that your pain is coming from the moving
parts and is not life-threatening or serious. The responses also allow you
to diagnose which movements are beneficial and which are harmful.

The exercise program consists of seven exercises: the first four
exercises are extension exercises (bending backward) and the last three
are flexion exercises (bending forward). *When beginning this exercise
program, you should stop any other exercises that you may have
been shown elsewhere or happen to do regularly; for example, for
fitness or sport.* If you want to continue with exercises, other than
those described in this book for low back problems, wait until your
pains have completely subsided. Note that some of the exercises in this
book are referred to as 'first-aid exercises'. These are helpful if you
have sudden attacks of back pain.

The purpose of the exercises is to abolish pain and, where appropriate,
to restore normal function – that is, to regain full mobility in the low
back or as much movement as possible. When you are exercising for
pain relief, you should move to the edge of the pain or just into the
pain, and then release the pressure and return to the starting position.
When you are exercising to regain lost movement or for stiffness, you
should try to obtain the maximum amount of movement; to achieve
this you may have to move well into the pain, which may also be felt
as a tight stretch rather than pain.

Postural correction and maintenance of the correct posture should always follow the exercises. For the rest of your life, whether or not you have back pain, good postural habits are essential to prevent the recurrence of your problems. Good posture also gives the added bonus of making you look healthier and more confident.

The intention is to correct any distortion or bulging that may have developed in the joints of the low back. By reducing the distortion or bulging of the intervertebral disc, the level of pain experienced can be reduced.

These exercises identify any movements or postures that are likely to increase distortion in the joints and delay recovery. This enables you to avoid damaging postures or activities in the future. If you can become pain-free and return to normal activities, your strength will return quite rapidly without any special extra effort.

Effect on Pain Intensity and Location

There are three main effects to look for while performing the exercises:

1. the exercises may cause the **symptoms to disappear**

2. they may cause an **increase** or **decrease** in the **intensity of the pain** that you experience

3. they may **cause the pain to move** from where you usually feel it to some other location.

In certain cases the symptoms first change location, then they reduce in intensity, and finally they cease altogether.

The effects of exercise on the intensity or location of pain can sometimes be very rapid. It is possible to reduce the intensity or change the location of pain after completing as few as ten or twelve movements, and in some conditions the pain can completely disappear.

In order to determine whether the exercise program is working effectively for you, it is important that you closely observe any changes in the intensity or location of your pain. You may notice that pain originally felt across the low back, to one side of the spine or in one buttock or thigh, moves towards the center of the low back as a result of the exercise. In other words, your pain localizes or *centralizes.*

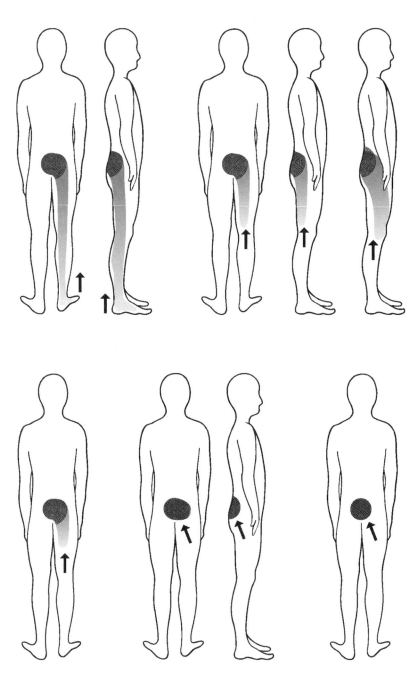

Figure 3) Progressive centralization of pain indicates suitability of exercise program

Centralization

Centralization is the movement of the pain to a more central location and centralization of pain (Figure 3) that occurs as you exercise is a good sign. If your pain moves to the mid-line of the spine and away from areas where it is usually felt, you are exercising correctly and this exercise program is the correct one for you.

The exercise that brings about a change of location or reduction in pain will, in most cases, be extension of the back. In these cases, extension becomes the ***mechanically determined directional preference,*** which is the movement in the direction that stops, reduces, or centralises pain.

The exercises in this book are the ones that most commonly match patients' directional preference. A few patients will not respond to extension exercises and these special cases must follow the instructions for other exercises where this is indicated in a later chapter.

The centralization of pain is the most important guide you have in determining the correct exercises for your problem. Research has demonstrated that if your pain centralizes or reduces on performing the exercises, your chances of rapid and complete recovery are excellent. Conversely, activities or positions that cause the pain to move away from the low back and perhaps increase in the buttock or leg are the wrong activities or incorrect positions and are a warning that you are at increased risk of damage if you persist with that particular exercise or posture.

Studies carried out independently in several countries in Europe and in the United States showed that ***centralization*** – movement of the pain to a more central location – and ***mechanically determined directional preference*** –movement in the direction that stops, reduces, or centralises pain – provide the most important guidelines for exercise prescription.

Perhaps the most important study was carried out in clinics, in several countries, staffed by clinicians trained in the McKenzie Method. It involved over 200 patients (Long *et al.* 2004). They were examined by health care clinician who determined which exercise centralized, reduced, or abolished their symptoms. The exercises were either flexion (bending forward) or extension (bending backward) as developed and described in my textbook for health care professionals, *The Lumbar Spine; Mechanical Diagnosis & Therapy*, published in 1981.

One-third of the patients were given the correct exercise based on directional preference, one-third were given the opposite exercise and one-third were told to keep generally active. After two weeks, over 90% using the directional preference exercise were better or resolved compared to 24% with the opposite exercise and 43% with general activity. Many of those patients who did the opposite exercise experienced a worsening of their condition. This is an important groundbreaking study that demonstrates that people with back pain respond best to different specific exercises, exactly as described in this book. It also demonstrates that if the wrong exercise is chosen, you can become worse.

The key to success is to let yourself be guided by the exercises that centralise, reduce or abolish your pain. To be certain of success, your pain must remain better after having completed the exercises. If it returns, it is likely that you have allowed your back to lapse into the wrong position or you have moved in the wrong direction. In this case you must perform the exercises once more, being very careful to maintain your lordosis when finished.

On commencing any of the exercises, an increase in pain is common and can be expected, as are new aches and pains in different places. As you continue to exercise, the pains should quickly diminish, at least to former levels. This usually occurs during the first exercise session and should be followed by centralization of pain. Once the pain no longer spreads outwards and is felt in the mid-line only, the intensity of the pain will decrease rapidly over a period of two to three days, and in anything from one to three or four weeks the pain should disappear entirely, provided you maintain good posture and continue exercising correctly.

If your low back pain is of such intensity that you can only move around with difficulty and cannot find a position in which to lie comfortably in bed, your approach to the exercises should be cautious and unhurried.

If your symptoms have been present continuously for many weeks or months, you should not expect to be pain-free in two to three days. The response will be slower but, if you are doing the correct exercises and being careful about your posture, it will only be a matter of ten to fourteen days before improvement begins. Remember, new exercises and new postures should cause temporary new pains.

If, following an initial pain increase, the pain continues to increase in intensity or spreads to places further from the spine, you should stop exercising and seek advice. In other words, do not continue with any of the exercises if your symptoms are much worse immediately after exercising and remain worse the next day, or if during exercising, symptoms are produced or increased in the leg below the knee.

The Exercise Program

Exercise 1: Lying Face Down

- lie face down with your arms beside your body and your head turned to one side (Exercise 1)

- stay in this position, take a few deep breaths, and then relax completely for two or three minutes. You must make a conscious effort to remove all tension from the muscles in your low back, hips and legs. Without this complete relaxation, there is no chance of eliminating any distortion that may be present in the joint.

This exercise is used mainly in the treatment of acute back pain and is one of the first-aid exercises for emergency back pain (see Chapter 9, Emergency Back Treatment). It should be done once at the beginning of each exercise session, and the sessions should be spread evenly six to eight times throughout the day until you go to bed at night. This means that you should repeat the sessions about every two hours. In addition, you may lie face down whenever you are resting.

This exercise is performed in preparation for Exercise 2.

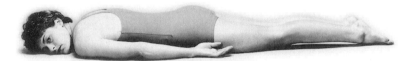

Exercise 1

Contents

Acknowledgements ii
About the Author iii

Introduction: *A Chance Discovery* vii

Chapter 1: *The Low Back or Lumbar Spine* 1
    Myths About Acute Back Pain 3

Chapter 2: *Understanding the Spine* 7
    Vertebrae and the Spine 7
    Functions of the Lumbar Spine 8
    Natural Posture 8
    Mechanical Pain 9
    Mechanical Low Back Pain 10
    Pain Location 12
    Self-Treatment 14
    When Self-Treatment Does Not Work 14
    Diagnosing Your Problem 14

Chapter 3: *Common Causes of Low Back Pain* 16
    Consequences of Postural Neglect 16
    Sitting 17
        Prolonged Sitting 18
    Posture and Sitting 18
        Sitting Correctly for Prolonged Periods 18
        Correction of the Sitting Posture 19
        How to Form a Lordosis Using the Slouch-Overcorrect
          Procedure 19
        Maintenance of the Lordosis 20
        The Lumbar Roll 20
        Regular Interruption of Prolonged Sitting 22
    Standing 23
        Prolonged Standing 23
        Correction of the Standing Posture 23
        Working in Stooped Positions 24
    Lifting 25
        Correct Lifting Technique 25
    Relaxing After Vigorous Activity 27
    Lying and Resting 28
        Correction of Surface 28
    Coughing and Sneezing 29

Exercise 2: Lying Face Down in Extension

- remain lying face down (2a)

- place your elbows under your shoulders so that you lean on your forearms (2b). During this exercise, as with Exercise 1, you should commence by taking a few deep breaths and then allow the muscles in the low back, hips and legs to relax completely. You should remain in this position for two to three minutes.

Exercise 2 is used mainly in the treatment of severe low back pain and is one of the first-aid exercises (see Chapter 9, Emergency Back Treatment). It should always follow Exercise 1 and is to be performed once per session. Should you experience severe or increasing pain on attempting this exercise, there are certain measures to be taken before you can continue exercising. These are discussed in the next chapter under 'No Response or Benefit'.

This exercise is performed in preparation for Exercise 3.

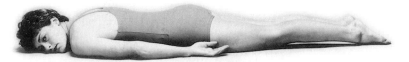

Exercise 2a

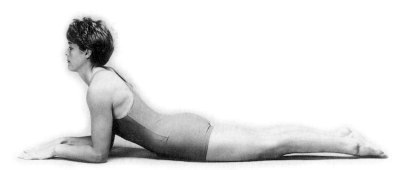

Exercise 2b

Exercise 3: Extension in Lying

This is the most useful and effective first-aid procedure in the treatment of acute low back pain. (see Chapter 9 Emergency Back Treatment). The exercise can also be used to treat stiffness of the low back and to prevent low back pain from recurring once you are fully recovered.

- remain lying face down (Exercise 3a) then place your hands under your shoulders in the press-up position (Exercise 3b). Now you are ready to begin.

A study from Denmark completed in 2002 (Larsen et al. 2002) looked at the value of the push-up type of exercise (Exercise 3) as recommended in this book. A group was given advice about back care from Treat Your Own Back *and then encouraged to do the exercise twice a day for a year. At the end of a year they were compared with a group who had not been doing the exercise (called a control group). The striking differences between the groups were in those who had a history of previous back pain episodes. The patients in the group who performed the exercise had half the number of recurrences of pain during the year compared with the group who did not exercise, and visits to the GP for back pain were a quarter of those who did not exercise. This study proves the value of* Treat Your Own Back *and of doing the push-up exercise regularly as a preventive measure.*

- as you straighten your elbows, push the top half of your body up as far as pain permits (Exercise 3c). It is important that you completely relax the pelvis, hips and legs as you do this, and remember to keep breathing normally

- keep your pelvis, hips and legs hanging limp and allow your low back to sag

- maintain this position for a second or two, then lower yourself to the starting position

- repeat this movement cycle in a smooth rhythmical motion and try to raise your upper body a little higher each time, so that in the end your back is extended as much as possible, with your arms as straight as possible (Exercise 3d)

- once your arms are straight, remember to hold the sag for a second or two as this is the most important part of the exercise. A more effective sag can be achieved by breathing all the way out while relaxing your low back, hips and legs. The sag may be maintained for longer than one or two seconds if you feel the pain is reducing or centralizing.

Never be satisfied that you have moved as far as possible. Say to yourself each time you push up, "further, further, further".

The exercise should be performed ten times per session and the sessions are to be spread evenly six to eight times throughout the day until you go to bed.

Should you not respond or have increasing pain on attempting this exercise, there are certain measures to be taken before you can continue exercising. These are discussed in the next chapter under 'No Response or Benefit'.

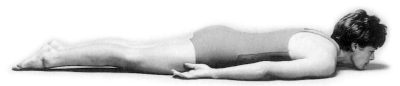

Exercise 3a

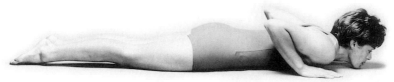

Exercise 3b

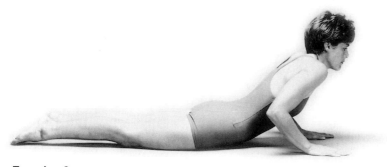

Exercise 3c

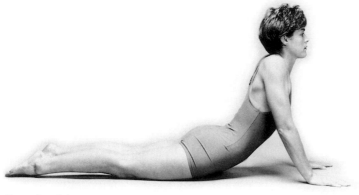

Exercise 3d

Exercise 4: Extension in Standing

- stand upright with your feet slightly apart, place your hands in the small of your back with the fingertips pointing backward so that they meet in the center of your spine (4a). You are now ready to begin.

- bend your trunk backward at the waist as far as you can, using your hands and fingers as a pivot point (4b). It is important that you keep the knees straight as you do this

- maintain this position for a second or two, and then return to the starting position

- repeat this movement cycle, and try to bend backward a little further each time so that in the end you have reached the maximum possible degree of extension.

When you are in acute pain, this exercise may replace Exercise 3 if circumstances prevent you from exercising in the lying position. This exercise, however, is not as effective as Exercise 3.

Once you are fully recovered and no longer have low back pain, this exercise is your main tool in the prevention of more low back problems. Whenever you find yourself working in a slouched or forward bent position, interrupt it regularly and perform Exercise 4 as a preventive measure, before pain appears or at the very first hint of pain.

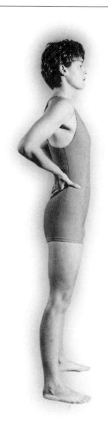
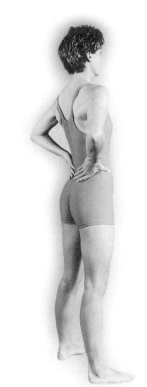

Exercise 4a

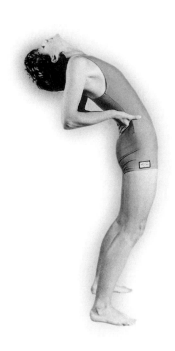
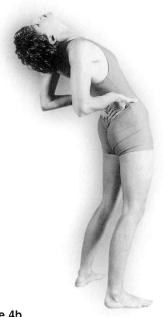

Exercise 4b

Exercise 5: Flexion in Lying

This exercise should be applied with caution as it could cause aggravation of your problem if commenced too soon.

- lie on your back (5a). Bend your knees with your feet flat on the floor or bed (5b). You are now ready to begin.

- bring both knees up towards your chest (5c)

- place both hands around your knees and gently but firmly pull the knees as close to the chest as pain permits (5d)

- maintain this position for a second or two, then lower the legs and return to the starting position. It is important that you do not raise your head as you perform this exercise or straighten your legs as you lower them

- repeat this movement cycle smoothly and rhythmically, and each time try to pull your knees a little closer to the chest so that in the end you have reached the maximum possible degree of flexion. At this stage your knees may touch the chest. Breathing out as you bring your knees to your chest makes it easier to perform this exercise and makes it more effective.

This exercise is used in the treatment of stiffness in the low back that may have developed since your injury or pain began. While damaged tissues may have now healed, they may also have shortened or contracted and become less flexible; it is now necessary to restore their elasticity and full function by performing flexion exercises. If you do not complete Exercises 5, 6, and 7 as described the contracted scar tissue may be at risk of tearing with any sudden forward bending. These exercises should be commenced with caution. In the beginning you must do only five or six repetitions per session, and the sessions are to be repeated three to four times per day. As you have probably realized, this exercise eliminates the lordosis once the knees are bent to the chest, so in order to rectify any distortion that may result, *flexion exercises must always be followed by a session of Exercise 3: Extension in Lying, or Exercise 4: Extension in Standing.*

You may stop performing Exercise 5 when you can readily pull the knees to the chest without producing tightness or pain. You may then progress to Exercise 6.

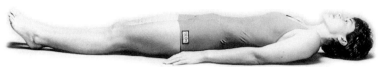

Exercise 5a

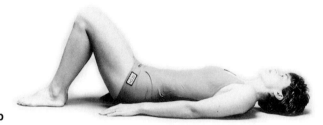

Exercise 5b

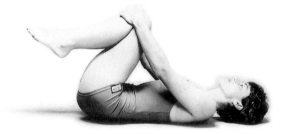

Exercise 5c

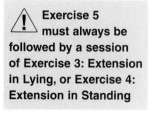

⚠ **Exercise 5 must always be followed by a session of Exercise 3: Extension in Lying, or Exercise 4: Extension in Standing**

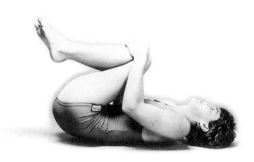

Exercise 5d

Exercise 6: Flexion in Sitting

- sit on the edge of a steady chair with your knees and feet well apart and let your hands rest between your legs (6a). You are now ready to begin.

- bend your trunk forward and touch the floor with your hands (6b)

- return immediately to the starting position

- repeat this movement cycle smoothly and rhythmically, and each time try to bend down a little further so that in the end you have reached the maximum possible degree of flexion and your head is as close as possible to the floor. The exercise can be made more effective by holding onto your ankles with your hands and pulling yourself down further (6c and 6d).

Exercise 6 should only be begun after the completion of one week of practice of Exercise 5, whether Exercise 5 has been successful or not in reducing your stiffness or pain. In the beginning you must do only five or six repetitions of Exercise 6 per session; the sessions are to be repeated three to four times per day and *must always be followed by Exercise 3 or 4.*

Exercise 6 must always be followed by a session of Exercise 3: Extension in Lying, or Exercise 4: Extension in Standing

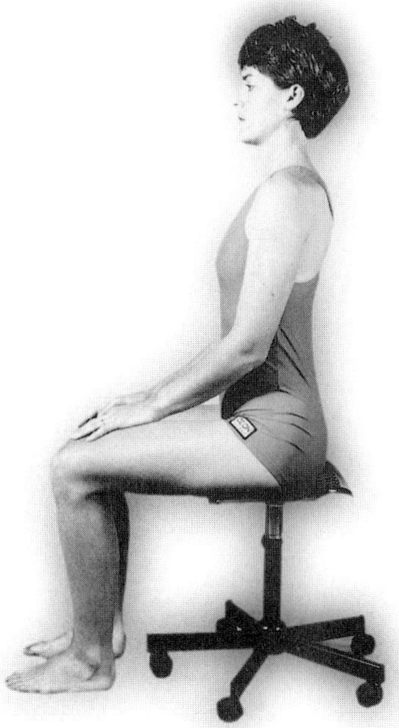

Exercise 6a

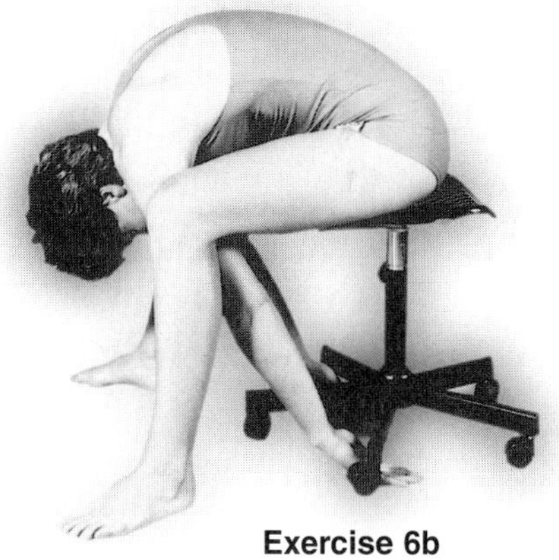

Exercise 6b

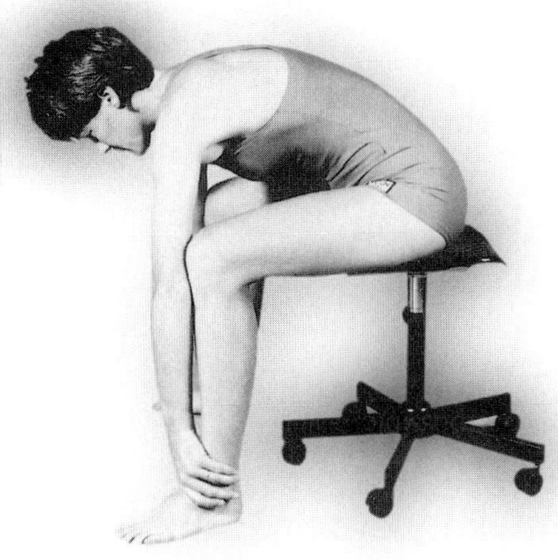

Exercise 6c

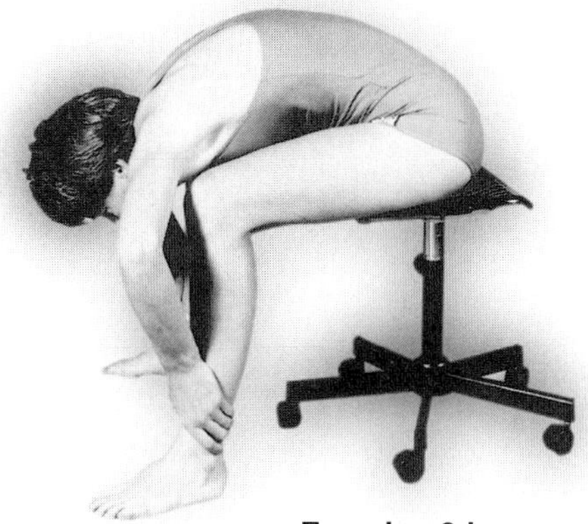

Exercise 6d

Exercise 7: Flexion in Standing

- stand upright with your feet well apart and allow your arms to hang loosely by your side (Exercise 7a). You are now ready to begin.

- bend forward and run your fingers down your legs as far as you can comfortably reach (Exercise 7b)

- return immediately to the upright standing position

- repeat this movement cycle smoothly and rhythmically, and try to bend down a little further each time so that in the end you have reached the maximum possible degree of flexion and your fingertips are as close as possible to the floor. Always return immediately to the upright standing position; do not remain bent forward.

Exercise 7 should only be commenced after the completion of two weeks of practice of Exercise 6, whether Exercise 6 has been successful or not in reducing your stiffness or pain. In the beginning you must do only five or six repetitions of Exercise 7 per session; the sessions are to be repeated once or twice per day and *must always be followed by Exercise 3 or 4.*

For a period of three months from the time you have become pain-free, Exercise 7 must never be performed in the first four hours of your day, during which time you are at more risk of recurrence.

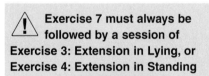

⚠ **Exercise 7 must always be followed by a session of Exercise 3: Extension in Lying, or Exercise 4: Extension in Standing**

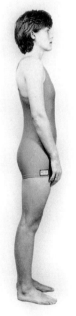

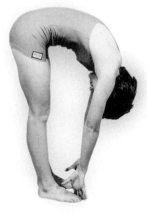

Exercise 7a   **Exercise 7b**

When to Apply the Exercises

You have probably experienced several acute or severe episodes of back pain in the past. You probably already know that the pain lessens over time. However, when you feel good, you, like all others with the same problem, tend to forget the precautions you should take. The main thing is to learn how the manoeuvres described here affect your particular back problem.

When You Have Significant Pain

Pain from an acute episode of low back pain is usually felt at all times, regardless of the position adopted or the movements being performed. With few exceptions, it is made much worse by sitting, or rising from sitting, and by bending forward. If the pain is also much worse on attempting to stand or walk and if you are unable to straighten up fully, it may not be possible for you to function and bed rest maybe the only alternative.

Research tells us that bed rest is not the best option for the treatment of acute and severe back pain and should be given for no more than two days. Those involved in that particular research study, however, would perhaps have a different view if they were to personally experience a severe bout of low back pain.

There are a few patients in severe pain who require longer than two days of bed rest before it is possible to get up and start moving around again. Nevertheless, early activity, exercise and movement are desirable for those forced to seek bed rest, and a determined effort to stand upright should be attempted at least once or twice every day.

You may commence the exercise program during this period of bed rest provided you can lie face down for short periods. You should perform Exercises 1 through to 3: Lying Face Down, Lying Face Down in Extension, and Extension in Lying. These exercises are first-aid for low back pain. Immediately following the exercises, roll onto your back and carefully insert the night Roll described on page 28 under the heading of 'Correction of Surface'. This maintains your back in the correct position during the period of bed rest.

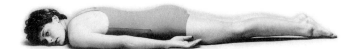

Exercise 1 — *Lying Face Down*

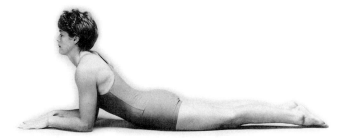

Exercise 2 — *Lying Face Down in Extension*

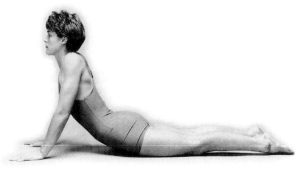

Exercise 3 — *Extension in Lying*

When to Start Exercising

Seek advice from your family doctor if the pain is of such severity that
it is impossible to perform any of the exercises or if it becomes
intolerable. Certain medications such as aspirin and non-steroidal
anti-inflammatory drugs (NSAIDS) may be necessary to provide
some respite from pain. Both these drugs have been found to be
the most useful for alleviation of acute back pain and have fewer
side effects than some other commonly prescribed medications.
Both have been recommended by the United States Federal
Government Agency for Health Care Policy and Research. If
your pain does not reduce or improve with these exercises,
immediately read 'No Response or Benefit', page 52.

As soon as you feel considerably better, no longer have constant
pain and are walking again – perhaps a day or two after you have
commenced exercising – you may stop Exercises 1 and 2, but
you should continue Exercise 3 and add Exercise 4: Extension
in Standing.

Exercise 4 —
Extension in Standing

About this time you should slowly introduce the slouch–overcorrect procedure (see How to Form a Lordosis on page 19), for you must now learn to sit correctly and maintain the lordosis just short of its maximum.

Once you no longer have acute pain, you should continue the exercise program as outlined in the following section.

When Acute Pain Has Subsided

For the past few days you have been doing Exercises 1 to 4 and have been maintaining a lordosis at all times. Once the distortion in the joints is reduced and any damaged tissue healed, it is necessary to restore your flexibility and recover your normal function. This is achieved by performing flexion exercises, which must be carried out in such a way that no further damage or tearing occurs within the recently healed soft tissues. The risks of further damage are much less when the low back is rounded in the lying position than in standing. Therefore you must now perform Exercise 5: Flexion in Lying.

Exercise 5 should begin when you have recovered from an acute episode of low back pain and have been pain-free for two to three days, even though you may still feel stiffness on bending forward. Exercise 5 may also be necessary should you have improved significantly with Exercises 1 to 4, but after two to three weeks still experience a small amount of pain in the center of the back that does not seem to disappear.

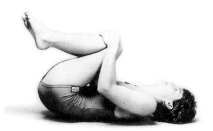

Exercise 5 — *Flexion in Lying*
to be followed by:

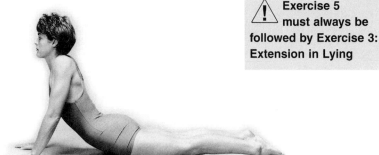

Exercise 3 — *Extension in Lying*

> ⚠ **Exercise 5
> must always be
> followed by Exercise 3:
> Extension in Lying**

It is not uncommon for some central, mid-line, and low back pain to be produced when starting with flexion in lying. An initial pain that wears off gradually with repetition of the exercise is acceptable; it means that shortened structures are being stretched effectively. **However, if flexion in lying produces pain that increases with each repetition, you should stop. In this case it is either too soon to start flexion or the exercise is not suitable for your condition.**

When you can touch your chest with the knees easily and without discomfort, you have regained full movement. You may now stop Exercise 5 and begin Exercise 6. After two to three weeks, Exercise 6 should cause no tightness or discomfort and once you have reached this point you may add Exercise 7 to your program. Exercise 7 should be carried out at the end of the day once or twice a week to ensure that all the soft tissues in the back remain extensible. After completing Exercises 6 and 7 you should follow the guidelines given to prevent recurrence of low back problems and continue with the exercise program as outlined below:

> ⚠️ **Exercise 5, 6 or 7 must always be followed by Exercise 3: Extension in Lying, or if that is not possible, Exercise 4: Extension in Standing**

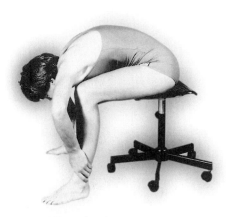

Exercise 6 — *Flexion in Sitting*

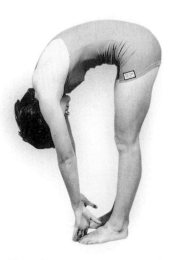

Exercise 7 — *Flexion in Standing*

To prevent recurrence of low back problems:

1.) perform Exercise 3: Extension in Lying on a regular basis, preferably in the morning and evening

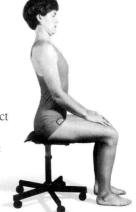

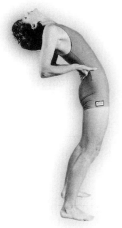

2.) perform Exercise 4: Extension in Standing at regular intervals whenever you are required to sit or bend forward for long periods. You should also do Exercise 4 before and after heavy lifting and during repeated lifting, and as soon as you feel minor strain developing in your low back

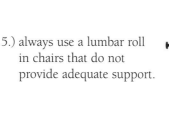

3.) practice the slouch–overcorrect procedure whenever you are becoming negligent about the correct sitting posture

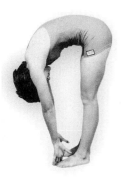

4.) perform Exercise 7 once or twice a week to remain fully flexible

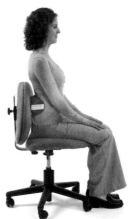

5.) always use a lumbar roll in chairs that do not provide adequate support.

It is advisable to exercise in the manner described above for the rest of your life, but it is a necessity that you develop and maintain good postural habits.

No Response or Benefit

If you have experienced no response or benefit from the exercises so far, it may be necessary to alter the way in which you apply the movements. Before doing so, however, ensure that you have not forgotten any of the basics outlined below:

- Did you feel better for a while after exercising only to find the pain returned later? If that is the case, you have probably missed some of the detailed advice.

- Did you push yourself up as far as possible, 'sagging' in the middle, when you applied Exercise 3?

- Did you say to yourself, 'Further, further, further' each time?

- Did you perform ten movements each time?

- Did you perform the exercises six to eight times per day?

- Did you stop all other exercise you may have been in the habit of doing?

- Did you bend over too far or for too long after exercising?

- Did you catch yourself sitting badly or without a lumbar roll at any time?

- Does your pain change its position and appear to move around? If so, you should follow the next section carefully.

If you are quite certain you have followed all the requirements listed above and are not improving, there are three or four more steps you can take that may abolish, reduce or centralize your symptoms.

The first step is to increase the pressure on your back as you perform Exercises 2 and 3. In some patients Exercise 3 gives a short period of relief, which is lost after an hour or two. This is usually because, although the direction of the exercise is the correct one, the force you can apply by yourself is insufficient.

The effectiveness of Exercise 3 can be improved by having another person apply pressure to your low back, which restrains your pelvis and increases the pressure at the low back. To do this, start by lying as for Exercise 1. Have your helper lean with both hands on your low back as shown by the therapist in. The pressure should be applied just at or slightly above the level of your pain. The intention is for you to press up as in Exercise 3 while your helper is applying the pressure to hold you down. This has the effect of accentuating the hollow in your back. It is vital that you allow your back to sag as this is proceeding. You should repeat this six or seven times, allowing the back to sink under the pressure of your helper as you try to push up.

The pressure applied by your helper should never cause severe pain that you cannot tolerate, or severely increase your pain. Each movement may increase your discomfort when you are pressed to the maximum, but this increase should stop when you return to the start position. If repeating this procedure is having the effect of gradually reducing your pain, you may repeat the exercise two or three times per day.

Adding this extra pressure may improve your condition rapidly and it may not be necessary to continue with this for more than a day or two. Under no circumstances should you continue with this extra pressure if you are uncertain about the effect it is having or if you have increased symptoms following the procedure.

How to Know if You Are Exercising Correctly

It is important that you read from the beginning of this chapter before starting the exercises to ensure that you fully understand the signs and symptoms you must look for while exercising. The exercises are of secondary importance to your complete understanding.

You are exercising correctly and in the right direction (mechanically determined directional preference) when:

- pain centralizes (moves from your leg, buttock or the side, towards the middle of your low back)
- pain intensity gradually decreases
- your range of movement increases

You are exercising incorrectly and in the wrong direction when:

- pain moves away from the spine
- pain intensity increases and remains worse
- your range of movement decreases

If your pain is moving away from the center of your back or radiating farther into your buttock and leg, you are moving in the wrong direction. Any exercise that is causing this should be stopped as soon as you are aware of the increasing intensity or spread of pain.

You now know how to perform the exercises correctly. However for you to be able to diagnose and treat your back problems successfully it is very important that you continue reading the rest of this book.

The second step is particularly important if your pain is felt only to one side of the spine, if it is felt much more to one side than the other or if it radiates into your buttock or leg. If your pain during the course of the day is felt only to one side, more to one side than the other, or if you feel pain more to one side as you perform Exercises 1, 2 or 3, you may need to modify your body position before commencing them.

To achieve this modification:

Step 1 adopt the position to perform Exercise 1 and allow yourself to relax for a few minutes

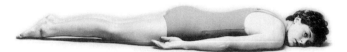

Step 1 *Lie face down relax.*

Step 2 remain face down and shift your hips away from the more painful side; that is, if your pain is usually more on the right side, you must move your hips eight or nine centimetres (three or four inches) to the left and once more completely relax for a few minutes

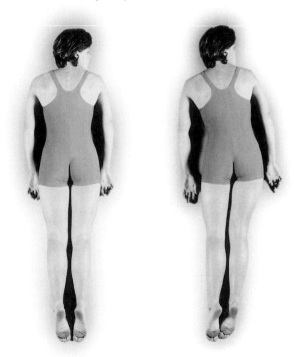

Step 2 *Move your hips away from pain.*

Step 3 while allowing the hips to remain off-center, lean on the elbows as described in Exercise 2, and relax for another three or four minutes. You are now ready to begin.

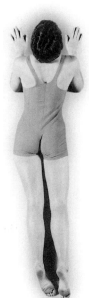

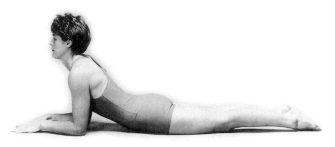

Step 3 *With hips off-center, lean on elbows.*

Step 4 with the hips still off-center, complete one session Exercise 3 and then relax once more.

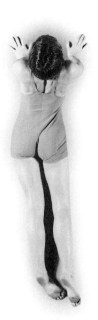

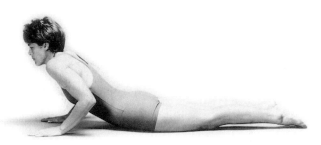

Step 4 *With hips off-center, you are ready to commence Exercise 3.*

You may need to repeat the exercise several times, but before each session of ten you should ensure that the hips are still off-center; remember, away from the painful side. It will be more difficult to push up in this position, but even with your hips in the off-center position, you should try with each repetition to move higher and higher. You should reach the maximum amount of extension possible, and your arms should be as straight as possible.

For the next three or four days you should continue to perform Exercises 1, 2 and 3 from the modified starting position. The frequency of the exercise and the number of sessions per day should be the same as recommended in the section 'When You Have Significant Pain', page 47.

After a few days of practice, you may notice that the pain is distributed more evenly across the back or may have centralized. Once this occurs, you may stop shifting the hips before exercising and continue exercises as recommended in the section 'When You Have Significant Pain', page 47. Occasionally shifting the hips away from the painful side is sufficient to stop the pain completely.

The third step is only for those people who have pain more to one side, or only to one side of the back, or who feel pain that is radiating into the buttock or leg.

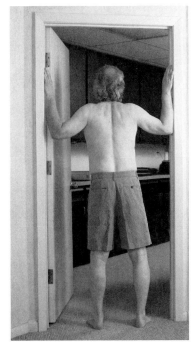
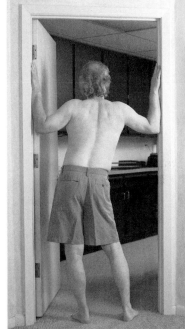

Step 1 *Stand in door way with hands and arms against the door frame*

Step 2 *Move your hips away from pain.*

- with correct standing posture, stand in the middle of a doorway with your feet about shoulder-width apart

- place the palms of your hands and forearms vertically against either side of the door frame

- using your arms against the doorframe to stabilise your upper body, move your pelvis and hips away from the side of pain.

- make sure you have gone as far as is tolerable then return your hips to the neutral start position.

The first movement or two may increase your pain and you may feel stiff and find it difficult to perform. You then repeat the movement gently eight to ten times, making sure you move your pelvis a little further with each repetition. As your movement improves, your pain should centralize or reduce. Once the pain has moved to and remains in the center of your back, return to Exercise 3.

Always remember that if your pain is moving away from the center of your back or radiating further into your buttock and leg, you are moving in the wrong direction. Any exercise that is causing this should be stopped as soon as you are aware of the increasing intensity or spread of pain.

If you continue to have pain that is not resolving, see the directory included at the back of the book for a clinician credentialled or diplomaed by the McKenzie Institute International.

Recurrence

Irrespective of what you are doing or where you are, at the first sign of recurrence of low back pain you should immediately start the exercises that previously led to recovery and follow the instructions given to relieve acute pain. You should at once commence **Exercise 4:** *Extension in Standing.* If this does not abolish your pain within minutes, you must quickly introduce **Exercise 3:** *Extension in Lying.* The immediate performance of Exercise 3 can often prevent the onset of a disabling attack. If your pain is already too severe to tolerate these exercises, you should commence with **Exercises 1 and 2:** *Lying Face Down and Lying Face Down in Extension.*

Finally, if you have one-sided symptoms that do not centralize with the exercises recommended so far, you should shift your hips away from the painful side before commencing the exercises and hold your hips in the off-center position while you exercise. In addition to the exercises, you must pay extra attention to your posture and maintain the lordosis as much as possible.

If this episode of low back pain seems to be different from previous occasions and if your pain persists despite the fact that you closely follow the instructions, see the directory included at the back of the book for a clinician credentialled or diplomaed by the McKenzie Institute International.

To obtain the names of Credentialed Members or Associates of the McKenzie Institute, see the Directory included at the back of the book.

When an Episode of Acute Low Back Pain Strikes

Immediately begin the self-treatment exercises. You must restore the lordosis slowly and with caution, never quickly or with jerky movements. You must allow some time for the distorted joint to regain its normal shape and position: a sudden or violent movement may retard this process, increase the strain in and around the affected joint and resulting in increased low back pain.

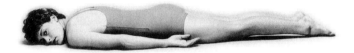

Exercise 1

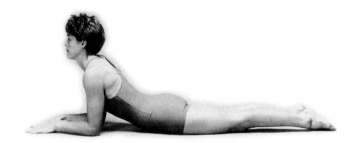

Exercise 2

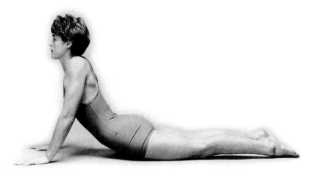

Exercise 3

When in acute pain you must, apart from exercising, make certain adjustments in your daily activities. These adjustments form a very important aspect of self-treatment. If you do not follow the instructions given below, you unnecessarily delay the healing process.

Sit as little as possible and for short periods only. If you must sit, choose a firm chair with a straight back, make sure that you have an adequate lordosis, and use a lumbar roll to support the low back. Avoid sitting on a low, soft couch, or with your legs straight out in front as in sitting up in bed or in the bath; both positions force you to lose the lordosis.

Many activities, such as vacuuming, brushing teeth, washing hands, washing dishes, working at a low bench-top etc can be modified adequately to enable maintenance of the lordosis:

- start with a good standing posture

- place your feet about shoulder width apart

- maintaining the lordosis, bend forward by moving your trunk forward at the hips, not at the waist or by rounding your upper spine

- if a workbench is too low, try standing with your feet a little further apart so your trunk is lower, minimizing the need to bend as far forward (at the hip).

If you have acute low back pain, ideally you should not lift at all. However, if you must lift, avoid objects that are awkward to handle or heavier than 15 kilograms (30 pounds). At all times you must use the correct lifting technique

If you are uncomfortable at night, you may benefit from a supportive roll such as an Original McKenzie® night Roll around your waist. For most people, it is recommended that the mattress should not be too hard but well supported by a firm base. If your bed sags, slats or a sheet of plywood between the mattress and base will level it, or else place the mattress on the floor.

When getting up from lying, keep your back in lordosis: turn on one side, draw both knees up, drop the feet over the edge of the bed, raise yourself to the sitting position by pushing your upper body up with your hands, and avoid bending forward at the waist.

Avoid coughing and sneezing while sitting or bending forward. If you feel a cough or a sneeze coming on, stand up immediately and bend backwards, placing your hands in your low back for support if necessary.

Avoid those positions and movements which initially caused your problems. You must allow some time for healing to take place.

Special
Situations

Treatment by REPEX (Repeated End-Range Passive)

Although the system of self-treatment that I have developed is effective
for most patients, the success of the method is sometimes limited
because of various factors that may prevent the patient from performing
the required movements.

Some patients may find that their pain is improving with the exercises,
but they cannot continue with them because of fatigue. Some are unable
to relax sufficiently when performing the push-up exercise. For the
exercise to be effective, it is vital that relaxation be obtained in the low
back. Others, especially the elderly, may have shoulder, elbow, wrist, and
even hip complaints that prevent them performing the key exercises.
Patients with certain disorders can have such restricted movement that
the self-treatment exercises are impossible to perform.

To overcome these difficulties, in 1986 I engaged an engineer to
develop a machine to provide controlled doses of specific repeated
movements to the low back. The machine, named REPEX, can
continuously move the low back many hundreds of times if necessary
without patient exertion.

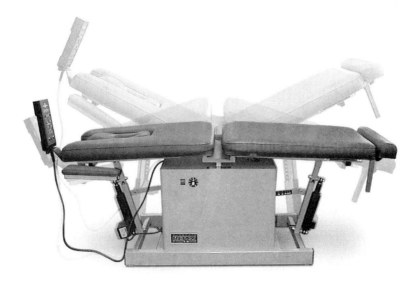

This form of treatment, known as continuous passive motion (CPM), has been found to improve the quality of repaired tissue and more rapid recovery when applied to injured joints of the body. REPEX is the first such machine to provide CPM for mechanical low back disorders.

If you have not resolved your back problem with the methods described in this book, perhaps REPEX could assist, particularly if you get relief after each session of exercise but the relief does not last. An increased number of movements may be all that is required to obtain lasting relief. Treatment by REPEX requires specialist expertise and is available only through diplomaed or credentialled members or associates of the McKenzie Institute.

Low Back Pain in Pregnancy

Both during and after pregnancy women are subjected to altered mechanical stresses that frequently result in low back problems. As the baby develops in the uterus, two simple changes take place that influence the mother's posture.

First, there is the gradually increasing bulk and weight of the developing baby. In order to maintain balance during standing and walking, the mother must lean further backward to counterbalance her altered weight distribution. The result of this postural adjustment is an increase in lordosis. In the final weeks of pregnancy, the lordosis may become excessive and this may lead to overstretching of the tissues surrounding the joints of the low back.

Second, to prepare the body for the impending delivery of the baby, the joints of the pelvis and low back are made more flexible and elastic by a natural increase of certain hormones. This greater elasticity means that the joints involved become more lax and are easily overstretched when subjected to mechanical strains.

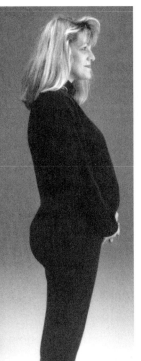

Typical standing position in pregnancy

After the child is born the mother is often too busy to care for herself properly, and sometimes the postural fault that has developed during pregnancy remains present for the rest of her life.

If your back problems commenced during or after pregnancy, it is likely that your lordosis has become excessive and your problems are caused mainly by postural stresses. If this is the case, the extension exercises recommended for the majority of people with low back pain are unsuitable for you at the present time, and you should concentrate mainly on correction of the standing

Good standing posture

posture. Problems caused by postural stresses are always resolved by postural correction. For one week, watch your posture closely. At all times you should maintain the correct posture, not only during standing but also while walking. You must stand tall, walk tall and not allow yourself to slouch. If after one week of postural correction the pain has disappeared or reduced considerably, faulty posture is to be blamed for your back problems.

For new mothers, bending forwards and lifting is usually unavoidable, however it is important that prolonged bending is avoided and correct lifting techniques (Page 25) are used. Good standing posture should be adopted immediately after any forward bending or lifting.

If your back problems commenced during or after pregnancy and you feel worse when standing and walking but much better when sitting, extension exercises again are not suitable for you. In addition to the postural correction in standing and walking, you should perform flexion exercises and self-treatment consisting of Exercises 5 and 6: Flexion in Lying and Flexion in Sitting.

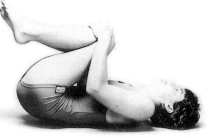

Exercise 5 —
Flexion in Lying

During the first week you should perform Exercise 5 ten times per session and six to eight sessions per day. When you have improved to some extent with this procedure, you should add Exercise 6 in the second week. Exercise 6 must follow Exercise 5 and should be done with the same frequency. Flexion exercises performed to relieve back pain appearing during pregnancy should not be followed by extension in lying. Once you are completely pain-free, you may stop Exercise 5. In order to prevent recurrence of low back problems, you should continue Exercise 6 twice per day, preferably in the morning and evening. At all times you should maintain good postural habits, but a lumbar roll should not be used in your case.

Exercise 6 —
Flexion in Sitting

If you are uncertain as to which of these two categories you belong, or if you do not respond to the flexion exercises, you should consult your family doctor or a therapist credentialled or diplomaed by the McKenzie Institute International.

Low Back Pain in Athletes

The symptoms of low back pain occurring in athletes can be confusing due to several factors. First, athletes are highly motivated to participate in their treatment and sometimes carry to excess the advice given to them in an attempt to speed recovery. This over-exuberant participation in their rehabilitation often delays rather than accelerates the healing process.

A second point is that the athlete's enthusiasm often encourages them to return to full participation long before healing is complete.

The third and certainly most common source of confusion stems from the common belief of athletes that their problem lies in their frequent participation in a particular activity, a belief that may be reinforced by a health care clinician. It is not difficult to reach this conclusion, for probably three out of five athletes who experience low back pain state that it appears after they have participated in sport or indulged in some equally vigorous activity.

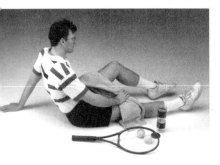

Slouched position after activity

The cause of pain is frequently the adoption of a slouched position following the thorough exercising of their joints. After exertion we usually sit down and relax. Because we are tired, the relaxed sitting posture is adopted almost immediately. In other words, after strenuous activity we collapse in a heap and slouch badly. During vigorous exercise, joints of the spine are moved rapidly in many directions over an extended period of time. This causes the soft tissues surrounding the joints to become thoroughly loosened and prone to overstretching when subject to inappropriate postures. In addition, the fluid gel content of the spinal discs can now be more readily displaced.

If low back pain has occurred as a result of participation in a particular activity, then recommending rest from that activity would be appropriate advice. However, if the pain has appeared after the activity has ceased and is a result of adopting a slouched sitting posture, such advice would be entirely inappropriate. To advise an athlete to cease participation in his favorite pastime can result in serious emotional and physical consequences.

If you are an athlete or if you participate in vigorous activities and have recently developed low back pain, it is necessary to expose the true cause in order to treat your condition correctly and successfully. It must be determined whether your pain appeared during the particular activity or whether it developed afterwards. If the pain appeared during the activity itself, then your sport may well be the cause of the present problems. You may remember something that happened at the time of the activity and can describe what you felt at that moment. However, numerous people who have back pain and participate in sport never feel discomfort or pain while they are participating or competing; their pain appears after the activity.

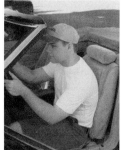

Slouched driving posture

It is easy to determine if your low back problems are the result of slouched sitting. From now on, immediately after activity, consider your posture carefully and sit correctly with the low back in moderate lordosis supported by a lumbar roll. For example, if you have completed a few sets of tennis, finished a round of golf or competed in a football or hockey game, you must not sink into a comfortable chair, sit slouched on the bench, or slouch in the car while you drive home. You must sit correctly with posture maintained meticulously. Should no back pain result from this extra postural care, the answer to your problem is clear and the responsibility for preventing further trouble is entirely your own.

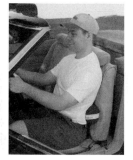

Good posture supported by a lumbar roll

If you fall into the group of people who develop pain *only* after activity, it is undesirable for you to begin the exercises at the same time as commencing the postural correction. If the exercises are performed in conjunction with postural correction, it is impossible to determine from which source the improvement was derived, so always work on postural correction first.

If your pain continues to appear after activity in spite of correcting your posture, it is possible that you have weakened or damaged some of the soft tissues in your low back. If this is the case, now is the time to commence self-treatment and you should perform Exercises 3 and 4: Extension in Lying and Extension in Standing on a regular basis.

Poor posture is often seen in athletes during intervals of non-participation, such as waiting to take the field in baseball, tennis, football, cricket or hockey. It is necessary to maintain good posture during these intervals. A conscious effort must also be made to maintain good posture after completion of the activity, when you are more likely to be physically tired and less likely to thinking about correct sitting posture.

If your pain appears regularly while running or jogging, you should commence the self-treatment program as outlined under the heading Emergency Back Treatment (Chapter 9) You should also seek advice regarding the type of footwear you use, the surface you run on and possibly your running technique. If your problems persist despite following the advice, you may need special treatment.

Low Back Pain in the Over 55

If you are over 55 or thereabouts, you may notice that you experience a more persistent ache in the low back, but no longer have the acute and severe episodes that affected you in your more active and vigorous days. It is now known that acute low back pain tends to occur less frequently once we pass this age. Nevertheless, this aching can cause significant problems, especially if you are forced to reduce activity. The human body thrives on activity and decays with prolonged inactivity. It is undesirable for any of us, irrespective of age, to reduce our levels of activity. Only if reduced activity is forced upon us by significant health problems should we exercise less.

You may also be told that you have degenerative changes in your back or that you have arthritis and have to live with these problems. While it may be true that your back has worn somewhat with ageing, it is certainly not true that you just have to live with the discomfort. It has been found that many people who have age-worn joints in their spines have never had back pain, and we now know that the wearing, in itself, is not a cause of pain.

There are few people who would not derive some benefit from the postural advice or the exercises, or both. Everyone over the age of 55 should carry out the advice regarding the correction of the sitting, standing and lying postures.

Not everyone in the older group will be able to perform all the exercises as advised, but all should try. I have found that age is not necessarily a barrier to the successful application of the exercises and, although there are some who may not succeed because of weakness or disability, most are able to advance at least partway through the recommended program.

My advice is to start by perhaps reducing the number of exercises to be performed at each session and to perform fewer sessions during the day. Do not hurry the process and always rest adequately after completing the exercises, properly supported in the correct position.

Osteoporosis

From middle-age many women are affected by a disorder called *osteoporosis*, which is essentially a mineral deficiency disorder. During and after menopause, there is a significant and continuing deficiency in calcium replacement that must often be supplemented with calcium on a regular basis. As a consequence of calcium deficiency there is a weakening of bone structure, resulting in a slow but progressive reduction in height. This allows the posture to become extremely rounded, especially in the middle or thoracic part of the spine.

In persons affected by this disorder, there are risks of fractures occurring without any significant forces being applied to the bones of the vertebrae. Research conducted at the Mayo Clinic in the United States has demonstrated that extension exercises performed regularly (Photo 7.6) had significantly reduced the number of compression fractures in the group exercising in this manner. A similar group exercising differently and a group not exercising at all had significantly more fractures when examined at least one year later. This study suggests that women from perhaps the age of 40 onwards should practice these extension exercises as described on a regular basis. My own recommendation would be repetitions of 15 to 20 times, four or five times per week. If you are uncertain regarding this advice, discuss the matter with your doctor before commencing the program. Should you have difficulties with the exercises, consult a health care clinician who will show you ways to modify the exercise without necessarily reducing its effectiveness.

The muscles strengthened by performing the exercises recommended by the Mayo Clinic study are also the muscles responsible for holding you upright, and it is probable that maintaining good posture at all times will assist in the strengthening process. This may also reduce the likelihood of small fractures occurring.

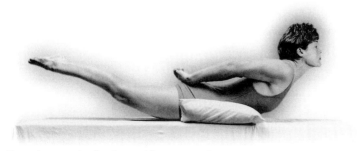

Extension exercise for those with osteoporosis

Common Remedies

Medication for Pain Relief

Most common back pains are mechanical in origin and therefore are affected only by drugs with pain-relieving capabilities. There are no drugs capable of removing the causes of common backaches and pains; therefore, medication should only be taken when your pain is severe.

Certain medications such as aspirin and non-steroidal anti-inflammatory drugs (NSAIDS) have been found to be the most useful for alleviating acute back pain and have fewer side effects than some other commonly prescribed medications. Both have been recommended by the US Federal Government Agency for Health Care Policy and Research.

Bed Rest

When your back pain is so severe that bed rest is required, this period of rest should be no more than two or three days at the most. A study conducted in the United States demonstrated that those patients resting in bed for two days recovered as well as those remaining in bed for seven days, in other words no benefit was gained from remaining on bed rest for any longer than two days. Those patients remaining mobile were able to go back to work sooner than those who rested for either two or seven days. Nevertheless, I have seen many patients who could still not arise from bed after ten days.

Acupuncture

Acupuncture may be able to relieve pain if all else has failed. The scientific evidence for its use is inconclusive and could not be recommended in national guidelines. Like taking medication, you may obtain relief from acupuncture, but acupuncture itself does not correct the underlying mechanical problem and certainly will not allow you to manage your own problem in the future. In fact, as with other passive therapies where a health professional 'does something to you', this procedure has the potential to create dependency.

Emergency Back Treatment

IN CASE OF A SUDDEN ONSET OF ACUTE PAIN, CARRY OUT THE FOLLOWING INSTRUCTIONS:

1. immediately lie face down. If this is impossible because of pain intensity, go to bed and attempt exercises the next day

2. if absolutely necessary, rest for two days maximum, correctly supported

3. use a rolled towel or an Original McKenzie® night roll around your waist when resting in bed

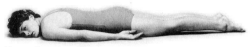

Exercise 1

4. perform Exercises 1, 2 and 3 ten times every two hours during your waking hours

5. if the pain is more to one side and not reducing, move hips away from the painful side and do Exercises 2 and 3

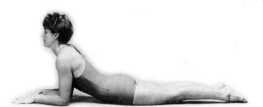

Exercise 2

6. avoid all movements that aggravate symptoms

7. do not slouch or bend forward for three to four days

8. use perfect posture at all times. Use a lumbar roll for support when sitting.

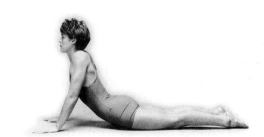

Exercise 3

References

Cherkin DC, Deyo RA, Battie M, Street J, Barlow W (1998). A comparison of physical therapy, chiropractic manipulation, and provision of an educational booklet for the treatment of patients with low back pain. NEJM 339.1021-1029.

Croft PR, MacFarlane GJ, Papageorgiou AC, Thomas E, Silman AJ. (1998). Outcome of low back pain in general practice: a prosepective study. BMJ 316.1356-1359.

Enthoven P, Skargren E, Oberg B. (2004) Clinical Course in Patients Seeking Primary Care for Back and Neck Pain. Spine 29.21

Koes BW, Bouter LM. Beckerman H, van der Heijden GJMG, Knipschild PG (1991). Physiotherapy exercises and back pain: a blinded review. BMJ 302.1572-1576.

Koes BW, Assendelft WJJ, van der Heijden GJMG, Bouter LM (1996). Spinal manipulation for low back pain. An updated systematic review of randomized clinical trials. Spine 21.2860-2873.

Kovacs, *et al.* (2003). Effect of firmness of mattress on chronic non-specific low-back pain: randomised, double-blind, controlled, multicentre trial. *The Lancet.* Nov. 15:362(9396):1599-1604.

Larsen K, Weidick F, Leboeuf-Yde C (2002). Can passive prone extensions of the back prevent back problems? Spine 27.2747-2752.

Long A, Donelson R, Fung T (2004). Does it matter which exercise? A randomized control trial of exercise for low back pain. Spine 29.2593-2602.

Udermann BE, Spratt KF, Donelson RG, Mayer J, Graves JE, Tillotson J (2004). Can a patient educational book change behaviour and reduce pain in chronic low back pain patients? Spine 4.425-435.

Williams, MM. Hawley J.4, McKenzie RA, van Wijmen PM (1991) A comparison of the effects of two sitting postures on back and referred pain. Spine 16, 1185-1191

The McKenzie Institute® International Center for postgraduate study in Mechanical Diagnosis and Therapy® (MDT)

The Institutes provides the only sanctioned training and certification in the McKenzie Method® of Mechanical Diagnosis and Therapy (MDT).

Enormous worldwide growth over the last decade has led The McKenzie Institute International to devise a regional alignment of its branches worldwide to better manage the overall educational programming and research as well as diversifying the conference programming and venues.

The 3 regions consist of Asia/Pacific and the Gulf States; Europe; and The Americas. Institute branches now exist in:

Americas - Brazil	Germany
Americas - Canada	Hellas/Cyprus
Americas – United States	Hungary
Australia	Italy
Austria /Switzerland	Japan
Benelux -	New Zealand
Belgium	Nigeria
Luxembourg	Norway
Netherlands	Poland
Croatia	Saudi Arabia
Czech Republic	Slovenia
Denmark	Sweden
Finland	United Kingdom
France	

Visit the Institute's website: http://www.mckenziemdt.org and select your country from the directory list for:

- the most current and comprehensive branch contact information

- find a certified McKenzie practitioner

Americas - United States

The McKenzie Institute® USA
Syracuse, New York
Tel: 1-315-471-7612, Toll-free 1-800-635-8380
Fax: 1-315-471-7636, E-mail: info@mckenziemdt.org

Americas - Canada

Robin McKenzie Institute Canada
Tel: Toll-free 1-800-463-8568
Email: mckenziecanada@bellnet.ca

The contact information is provided for the purpose of verification of certified MDT practitioners and arranging an office visit for an appropriate patient evaluation with that practitioner. It is not advisable for the patient or the practitioner to discuss or dispense treatment recommendations over the telephone.

Due to various country laws, not all branches will be able to provide web listing of their certified practitioners. If a country is not listed in our Branch & Therapist Locator, contact the branch in question directly for more details on whether any certified practitioners are available in that country.